What's Eating Our Kids?

A PARENT'S GUIDE to FOOD ALLERGY, INTOLERANCE, AND TOXICITY

JULIE A. WENDT, MD

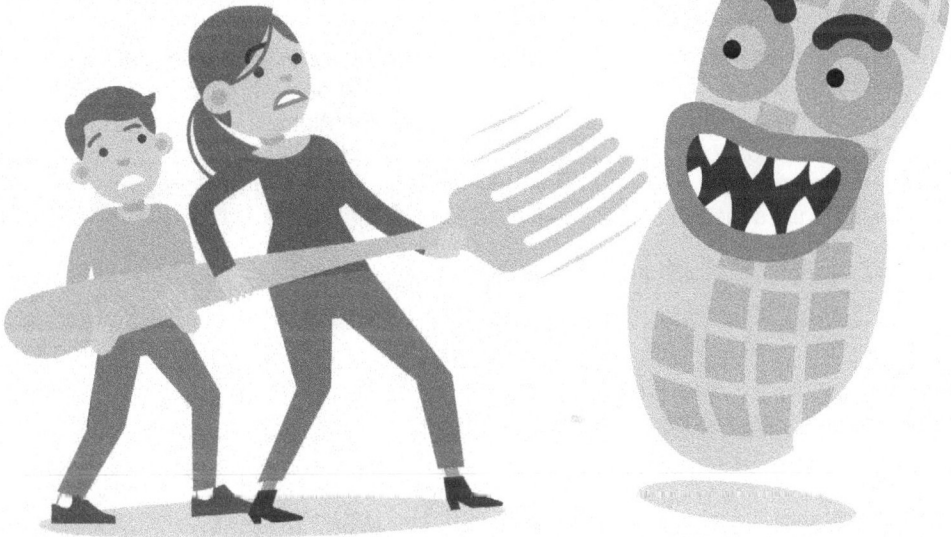

Publishing support provided by
Ignite Press
5070 N. Sixth St. #189
Fresno, CA 93710
www.IgnitePress.us

ISBN: 979-8-9875600-0-6
ISBN: 979-8-9875600-1-3 (Hardcover)
ISBN: 979-8-9875600-2-0 (E-book)

For bulk purchases and for booking, contact:

Julie Wendt
Bulk purchases - www.relieveallergyaz.com/book
Booking - bookjulie@relieveaz.com

Because of the dynamic nature of the Internet, web addresses or links contained in this book may have been changed since publication and may no longer be valid. The content of this book and all expressed opinions are those of the author and do not reflect the publisher or the publishing team. The author is solely responsible for all content included herein.

This book is not meant to substitute for medical care by an allergist-immunologist nor is it intended to provide medical advice or imply a Physician-Patient relationship with its readers or their children. It is intended to provide guidance, direction, and moral support from someone who has been on almost every side, patient, physician, and patient's parent, of food allergies. This is also not meant to be a "do-it-yourself" manual or a "how to" overcome your child's food issue. Some of the issues mentioned, whether food allergy or a look-a-like, can be dangerous or if left unchecked, deadly. Please develop a relationship with a Physician you trust to help you with diagnosis, advice, questions, and treatment regarding your child's medical conditions.

Library of Congress Control Number: 2023900031

Cover design by Marty Harris, Marty Harris Illustration
Content editing by Bonnie McDermid, Wordsmith.Ink
Copy editing by Elizabeth Arterberry
Illustrated by Marty Harris, Marty Harris Illustration
Interior design by Eswari Kamireddy

FIRST EDITION

F1

WHAT PEOPLE ARE SAYING ABOUT
WHAT'S EATING OUR KIDS?

What's Eating Our Kids? is a comprehensive, yet easy to "digest," explanation of food allergy, intolerance, and toxicity in children. Dr. Wendt has accurately summarized the science of food immunology into an engaging book that is sure to help many families as they navigate the complexities of feeding children with underlying medical issues. I plan to keep a copy of this book in my office and recommend it to my patients, who are always seeking reliable sources of medical information.

—Sakina S. Bajowala, MD
Founder and Medical Director of Kaneland Allergy and Asthma Center,
author of *The Food Allergy Fix*

Dr. Wendt's book is an entertaining, easy-to-read food allergy primer for those dealing with any food-related issues. It gives specialized insight from a board-certified Allergist-Immunologist and also from the personal perspective of an "allergy mom." As a person who cares passionately about food and believes it to be a central focus in many people's lives, I also see Dr. Wendt's similar passion manifested in this book.

—Stanley Cheng, DO
Allergy and Immunology Fellow
University of Buffalo, Buffalo, New York

I really enjoyed reading your book, Dr. Wendt. It is comprehensive and accurate and will serve as an excellent bridge between professionals and laypeople. Parents and families will be greatly benefitted by reading this book. Your explanation of food allergy versus food intolerance is very useful, as are the many real stories you share from your family's and professional experience as an Allergy-Immunology doctor.

—Hirohito Kita, MD
Professor of Immunology and Professor of Medicine at Mayo Clinic,
Scottsdale, AZ and Rochester, MN Professor of Medicine,
Mayo Clinic College of Medicine, Rochester, MN

Dr. Wendt has written a comprehensive book that provides useful information not just about health problems triggered by foods but also about the associated disorders that disrupt the lives of millions. It provides an insider's look at the evolving theories and practices of the most forward-thinking Allergist-Immunologists in the United States and around the world in the field of food allergies and intolerances. *What's Eating Our Kids?* demonstrates the determination and passion Dr. Wendt and I share to help our patients live normally in spite of food allergy, intolerance, and toxicity. The education and encouragement readers will receive through this book will, undoubtedly, improve the health of many patients and their families.

—R. L. Wasserman, MD, PhD
Medical Director of Pediatric Allergy and Immunology
Medical City Children's Hospital, Dallas, Texas

Dr. Wendt is being too humble calling this a guide; she's written an encyclopedia covering the field of food allergy and beyond. Whether it is read cover to cover or used as a reference to solve a reader's particular problem, this book will be treasured by all. The author's caring and passionate nature—what every patient hopes to find in their doctor—oozes out from every page as she shares her personal stories and sage advice. A must-read for food allergy families.

—Hugh H. Windom, MD
Founder and Medical Director of Sarasota Clinical Research,
Clinical Professor of Medicine at the University of South Florida,
Department of Medicine, Division of Allergy and Immunology

*To my parents, Al and Diane, who are the most amazing people in the world.
I love you so much. You are the perfect parents. I still look up to you.*

*To my husband, Phil, the love of my life and soulmate, and to my children, Katie,
Alex, Brigham, Bronson, Bridge, Kately, and Brice. Each of you is very important to
me and I love you dearly. Katie and Alex, everything I do is dedicated to and for you.*

*And to my patients: I pray that I have always taken good care of you
and that you felt loved and important in my care.*

Acknowledgments

I would like to express my gratitude to my mentors. First, Dr. Edward Voss of the University of Illinois, my first Immunology professor, who was the best teacher I have ever had in my life and who instilled the joy of learning immunology in me. This was imperative because immunology is a constantly evolving field.

Drs. Anita Gewurz, Giselle Mosnaim, James Moy, and Mary Tobin of Rush University Medical Center were the most amazing clinical mentors ever. I learned so much from all of you, perhaps most importantly how to think about clinical problems and stand on my own two feet as a physician.

I am grateful to my parents for their love, prayers, caring, and sacrifices to ensure I had the best education possible. I am extremely grateful to my husband, who is my greatest source of all love and support in this project as well as in my career. I have always said I love my work as an allergist so much I'd do it even if I didn't get paid, because I adore my patients so much. But my husband is the one who has made this possible during the times when I was not paid for my work as a physician while opening and growing my practice.

Dad, I still remember the times you spent with me, sparking my interest in biology, anatomy, and medicine. Most people go through life looking for a mentor, a teacher, to help them along the way. How fortunate was I to be born to one! You took every opportunity to teach, such as the lobster anatomy lesson in the restaurant on our East Coast trip, your lessons on the anatomy and function of plants (and the follow-up testing), and especially reviewing the guts of the see-through anatomy model and pointing out all the organs while shaving. You are an amazing Dad and I love you dearly.

Special thanks to my children Katie and Alex, for their love, understanding, and support through my long hours of work and writing, which sometimes limited our time together. Also, many thanks to my brother, Al, and my sister, Laura, for being my great supporters.

Thank you to the following amazing people who took the time to review my book and make comments. I admire each and every one of you for your great knowledge and individual perspective: Dr. Sakina Bajowala, Dr. Stanley Cheng, Gary Falcetano, Dr. Hirohito Kita, Alison Marshall, Darlene Trogani, Dr. R. L. Wasserman, and Dr. Hugh Windom. Mr. Falcetano is my dear friend and an expert on allergy testing, having worked at Thermo Fisher for many years.

Dr. Wasserman, Dr. Kita, Dr. Bajowala, Dr. Windom, and Dr. Cheng are stars in the field of food allergy. All have dedicated their lives to research in food allergy and are my heroes as well. I credit Dr. Wasserman, Dr. Bajowala, and Dr. Windom with bringing food oral immunotherapy into the mainstream of allergy/immunology practice and Dr. Cheng for his diehard drive to learn and perpetuate this amazing skill. All of these brilliant physicians speak regularly at events and even educate allergists at our national meetings. Dr. Kita is also a leader in food allergy and immunology research. Slowly but surely, more and more allergists are becoming comfortable with this therapy through their generous contribution of time and effort.

As a result of these long-term efforts by many allergist-immunologists to standardize and mainstream Food Oral Immunotherapy Treatment (FOIT), many food allergy patients are now able to better cope with, manage, and whenever possible, overcome their reactions to food. (See Chapter 5 for more information.)

Thank you to GlaxoSmithKline (GSK) for allowing use of the C-ACT test. GSK is a pharmaceutical company that has been dedicated to improving the lives of patients with allergies and asthma for many years. Thank you to Monash University for allowing use of its FODMAP application graphics. Monash University, through research and the FODMAP application, has revolutionized the lives of many patients. They have also been kind enough to review the chapter in which their work appears and make very helpful comments and suggestions.

Finally, thank you to my amazing editor, Bonnie McDermid, who, despite the great effort this book took, made editing fun and taught me about writing. That said, I would still rather just chat with her. Thanks are also due to Marty Harris and Amy Vince for their amazing artwork. You have all given me great joy as you made my concepts more accessible. Together, we made quite the team.

Contents

Foreword

Allergist-immunologists (allergists for short) must be medicine's sharpest detectives. Unlike detectives on television and in the movies, the allergist-detective's focus is not limited to a single event and the potential suspects include the whole panoply of human health and disease.

Although the word allergy (from the German word, *allergie*, which, in turn, was derived from the Greek word *allos*, meaning "other, different, strange") was coined in 1906 to describe reactions to external substances, today the word allergy is often used as an explanation for almost anything that goes wrong in the body. This means that the allergist may see a patient with a set of complaints he or she attributes to an allergic reaction when, in fact, the complaints are not manifestations of allergy at all but represent another disease altogether.

The challenge of sorting through the information to come to the correct diagnosis is one of the most stimulating things about being an allergist—and arriving at the right diagnosis that leads to a life-altering treatment is one of the most satisfying.

About 100 years after the first food-allergic child was treated with food oral immunotherapy (FOIT), allergists in the U.S. who recognized the huge burden borne by children and families with food allergies began trying to desensitize food allergy patients in the private allergy office.

The early adopters of this treatment shared their experiences and procedures with other board-certified allergists as more and more private allergy practitioners began to offer this treatment outside of clinical research studies. These early adopters also fostered the development of a community of private practice, creating a group of board-certified allergists who meet annually to exchange information about their FOIT procedures and their observations about how their patients respond. These meetings have produced several peer-reviewed publications and have advanced the practice of food allergy treatment for the benefit of patients and their families. This meeting is entirely supported by FOIT physicians without the participation of pharmaceutical companies, academic institutions, or allergy societies.

In addition, private food allergy practitioners have formed a Google Group to facilitate real-time communications about patient problems as they occur. By 2019, members of this Google Group had treated more than 15,000 food-allergic patients. Much of the information about food allergy discussed in this book is derived from this community of private practice board-certified allergists, of which Dr. Wendt is an active member and contributor.

Dr. Wendt has written a comprehensive book that provides useful information not just about health problems triggered by foods but also about the associated disorders that disrupt the lives of millions. It provides an insider's look at the evolving theories and practices of the most forward-thinking allergist-immunologists in the United States and around the world in the field of food allergies and intolerances.

What's Eating Our Kids? demonstrates the determination and passion Dr. Wendt and I share to help our patients live normally in spite of food allergy, intolerance, and toxicity. The education and encouragement readers will receive through this book will, undoubtedly, improve the health of many patients and their families.

R. L. Wasserman, MD
Dallas, Texas
January 12, 2023

Introduction

We never saw it coming. After eating fish for school lunch, as she had many times before, my sister Laura had a severe anaphylactic attack—shortness of breath, wheezing, chest tightness, swelling of her throat, flushing, itching, and hives.

Laura said this was the most frightening experience of her life. She struggled so hard to breathe, she wasn't sure she would survive until the paramedics arrived and took her to the hospital. (Frankly, it was extremely hard on the rest of the family, too, until we knew she was going to be fine.)

Thankfully, Laura recovered with excellent medical care and learned to manage her allergies, changing a lot of things for her and our whole family. For instance:

- Laura was tested by an allergist who later educated Laura and our family about ways to avoid another anaphylactic reaction.
- Laura never ate fish again. Whenever fish was served at home, Mom cooked Laura a different entrée.
- Shortly after Laura's fish allergy was discovered, we learned she was also allergic to bananas.
- Laura carried an epinephrine injector pen with her from that day forward.
- Our whole family and close friends learned what to do if Laura had another anaphylactic reaction.
- Today Laura "tests" foods to see if there is fish in them by touching them to her tongue, because her tongue itches and tingles in response. As her sister, I certainly believe her. However, as a board-certified allergist-immunologist, *I definitely do not recommend relying on this or any other self-testing method*!
- Discovery of your own or a family member's allergy is rarely this scary because the vast majority of allergic and non-allergic food reactions are mild. Only 1-2% are severe—like my sister's anaphylactic attack—and very few of those are fatal. There are only about 30 deaths from food allergy in the U.S. each year. (CDC)
- Laura's allergic reaction was one of several experiences that ultimately led me to become an allergist-immunologist. Now, after two decades of testing and treating many asthma, allergy, and hives patients, conducting research, and studying new methods and treatments, I have adopted state-of-the-art

treatments for food allergies, intolerances, and toxicity. We allergists who follow these protocols have helped thousands of allergy sufferers feel much better and live symptom-free the vast majority of the time. Our treatment approach has led to a paradigm shift in the lives of my patients and their families.

Your Child _Can_ Live a Normal Life with Allergies

It's true: an allergy diagnosis does not mean that life as you know it is over. I've had the satisfaction of guiding thousands of my patients and their families to much better health. No, your lives won't be the same, but you can learn what it takes, as many other allergy parents have. You will need new information—much of which you can find in this book—heightened vigilance, expert medical guidance, and cooperation from family, friends, and teachers.

Once you learn what you need to know and apply it, new habits will be formed, and your stress level will drop appropriately. While you will always stay vigilant, you and your child will no longer need to be fearful of navigating a world filled with allergy triggers.

I know because I've been there—I'm an allergy mom, too. My daughter has had asthma and allergies since she was 12 years old, and my son was also allergic; he had eczema triggered by soy and milk and reactive airway disease with wheezing after every viral infection. He's now outgrown these reactions. As a result, I have firsthand experience of the stresses, fears, and challenges allergy parents face, but I got through it and am confident you can too.

That's why I wrote this book—to pass along essential information that will increase your child's ability to lead a normal life.

Don't Go It Alone

You will need professional medical advice and guidance to manage your allergies and reactions, as well as those of family members. I urge you to seek out and work with a _board-certified_ allergist-immunologist because the most complex and serious allergic reactions are caused by the immune system. Therefore, it is to your great benefit to work with a physician who has a thorough understanding of the immune system and is also an expert at diagnosing and treating the entire spectrum of allergic and non-allergic reactions. Your allergist-immunologist will conduct the necessary allergy testing, determine your diagnosis, draw up a course of treatment, and guide you and your child through the treatment process.

If you have trouble selecting an allergist-immunologist, ask your family doctor or pediatrician to recommend someone to you. Ideally, your family doctor will partner with your allergist-immunologist to provide the medical information and guidance you need.

What It Takes to Become an Allergist-Immunologist

An allergist-immunologist (commonly referred to as an allergist) is a physician who is specially trained to diagnose, treat, and manage allergies, asthma, and immunologic disorders, including primary immunodeficiency disorders. These conditions range from the very common to the very rare, span all ages, and encompass various organ systems.

In the United States, becoming an allergist-immunologist requires at least an additional nine years of training beyond a bachelor's degree. After completing medical school and graduating with a medical degree, physicians undergo three years of training in Internal Medicine or Pediatrics, then pass the exam of either the American Board of Internal Medicine (ABIM) or the American Board of Pediatrics (ABP). Following that, becoming an allergist-immunologist requires at least two additional years of study, called a fellowship, in an Allergy/Immunology training program.

Those allergist-immunologists listed as ABAI-certified have successfully passed the certifying examination of the American Board of Allergy and Immunology (ABAI). Many of these individuals have achieved the rank of Fellow within the American Academy of Allergy, Asthma, and Immunology (AAAAI) and the American College of Allergy, Asthma, & Immunology (ACAAI). When you see FAAAAI and FACAAI alongside the designation of Medical Doctor, you know your allergist-immunologist has met many of the highest standards, stayed current on the most important and latest research and literature, and demonstrated leadership in the field.

How to Get the Most Out of This Book

What's Eating Our Kids? will help you better understand your child's or your own diagnosis, know what to expect during testing and treatment, give you practical tips on managing the allergy or intolerance, and guide you through the learning curve of your new role as a vigilant allergy patient or parent.

I wrote this book to be adjunct to the professional medical care you're getting and recommend you share it with your family doctor and your allergist-immunologist.

◆ ◆ ◆

No Room for Error

Prior to working in Allergy and Immunology, I was in an Internal Medicine residency. One day, while making rounds in the intensive care unit, a young lady of about 17 years of age was brought in, her face horribly swollen and nearly unrecognizable. As she wasn't able to breathe by herself, the medics had placed a tube down her throat and into her windpipe to give her oxygen.

I was told she had been dining in a restaurant when she accidentally ingested fish, despite being assured there was no fish in her food. But clearly, there was enough cross-contamination to set off a severe allergic reaction.

The paramedics struggled a long time to get control of her severely swollen airway. Tragically, she was already brain dead by the time she was admitted and transported to the intensive care unit. There, she declined until she passed away.

I will never forget this young woman. Her face is burned into my memory and will be forever, because an infinitesimally small amount of fish accidentally contaminated her dinner and caused her to die well before her time.

The moral of this true story: educate yourself (and your child if they are old enough to understand) and _never_ count on strangers to know better than you do.

Let's face it: some people are very respectful of others and some people are know-it-alls who insist their prejudicial beliefs are absolutely correct. Others just do not care, which I find saddest of all. In any case, make certain you understand whether or not a person has concrete knowledge of food allergens before you trust them with your own or your child's health and life. This book is intended to empower you in this way.

◆ ◆ ◆

Part 1: Allergy Basics

Chapter 1

Allergies & Other Reactions

What's Essential to Know about Your Family's Reactions to Food, The Environment, and Sensitizing Substances

Chapter Preview

- What is a reaction?
- What is the difference between an allergic reaction and a non-allergic reaction?
- How to distinguish between seasonal allergies, food allergies, intolerances, and look-alike reactions.
- Which allergies and reactions are of greatest concern to the affected person and their family members.
- Which symptoms to look for, how to respond, and when to get medical attention.

Chapter Introduction

What Is a Reaction and What Are the Different Types of Reactions?

First, a reaction is the body's response to a substance called a trigger.

Second, reactions are either allergic or non-allergic. Allergic reactions like hay fever and anaphylaxis are caused by the body's immune system. Non-allergic reactions are caused by a physiological intolerance, exposure to a toxic substance or various chemicals, or an internal metabolic process.

Third, let's clarify the different types of reactions so you understand which reactions are of the greatest concern, whether or not it's likely the patient can outgrow or overcome the reaction, and help you know when self-care is enough or professional medical care is needed.

Comparison of Food Allergy, Intolerance, and Toxicity

1. Allergic (mild to severe)
2. Intolerance
3. Toxicity (unknown)
4. Other (e.g. chemical, metabolic)

Percent of Patients Affected by Food Allergies, Intolerance, and Toxicity

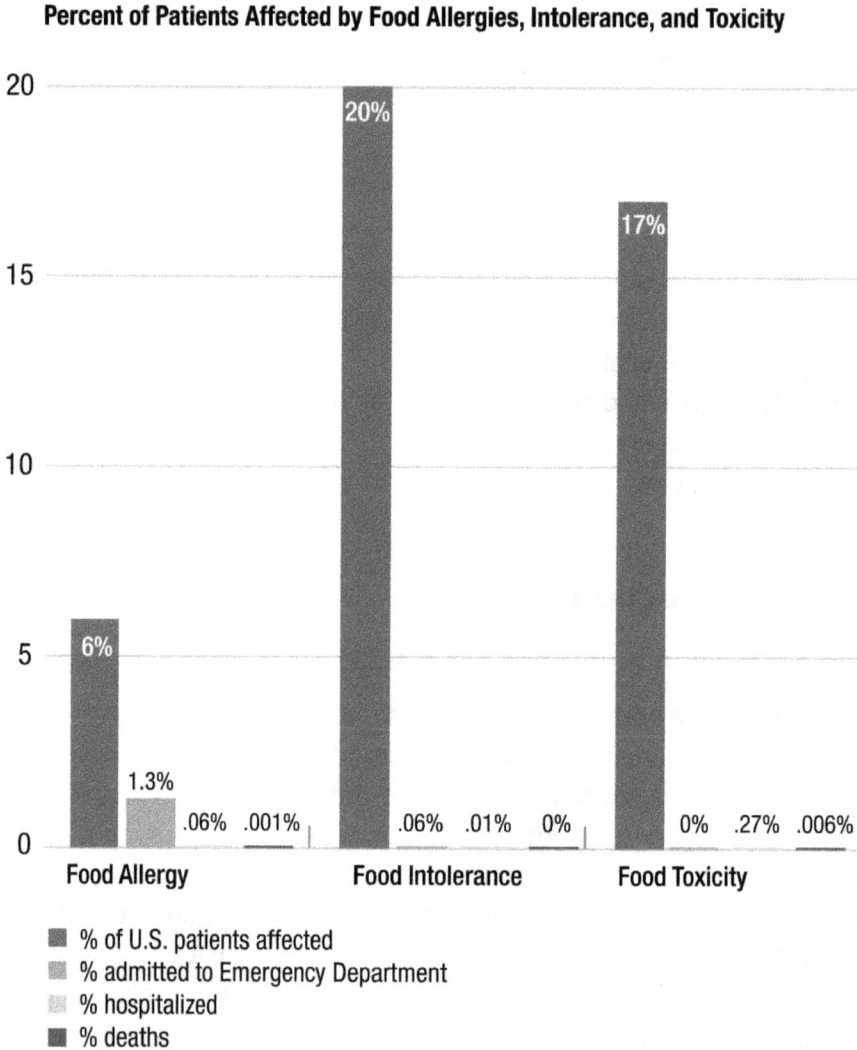

Figure 1: While many people believe they have allergies, the actual number of patients with allergies is much smaller than the number of those who have food intolerance and food toxicity.

ALLERGY
SYMPTOMS

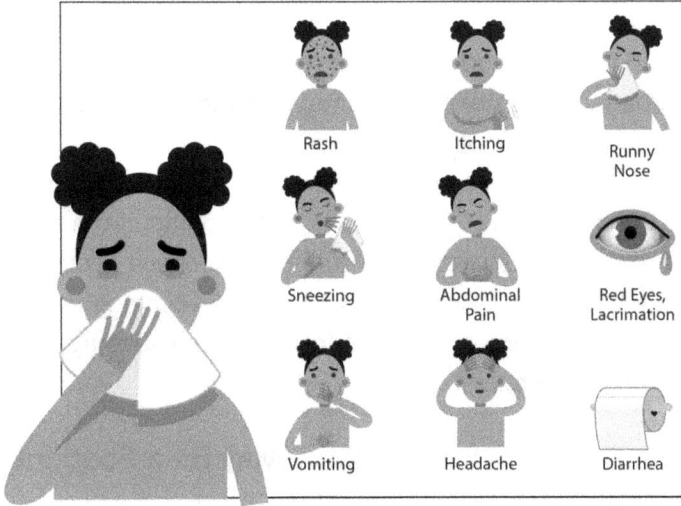

ALLERGY
TRIGGERS

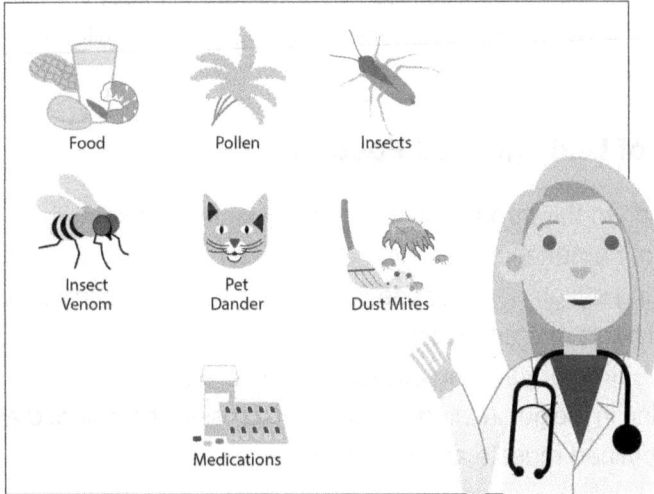

Figure 2: Symptoms and triggers of allergy.

Reactions Can Be Triggered by a Range of Substances

While this book is primarily concerned with reactions to food, it's important to understand that insect bites, latex, drugs, pollen, and other substances can also trigger reactions, some of which can be life-threatening.

Many Reactions Have Look-Alike Symptoms

Visible symptoms of reactions can range from mildly bothersome to life-threatening. For example, diarrhea, abdominal pain, and nausea can signal food intolerance (such as lactose intolerance) or a food allergy. However, if those symptoms escalate to swelling of the throat and breathing problems, a severe food allergy may be in play and anaphylaxis may be the result.

Since both allergies and intolerances can cause nausea and digestive distress after eating, what's the difference? Whereas an upset stomach from a food intolerance will be over after the food has passed through the digestive system, a true allergic reaction to a food could escalate into a serious medical emergency. No, not all food allergies are severe, but the potential exists for increasing severity over time and escalating symptoms during a reaction.

What You Might Think Is a Food Allergy May Be a Food Intolerance

About 26 million (11%) of American adults have been diagnosed with a food allergy. Around 19% of U.S. adults *believe* they are allergic to certain foods when it's more likely they have a food intolerance (Gupta 2019). After years of observing and treating patients, I believe these statistics do not adequately reflect the great number of people who suffer for years from undiagnosed allergies *and* intolerances, simply because they don't know help is available.

Symptoms of Undiagnosed Food Allergies:

- Swelling in the throat, which can feel like having something stuck there
- Itching, numbness, and tingling on the face and around the mouth
- A feeling of lightheadedness caused by a decrease in blood pressure
- Rapid heart rate and increased anxiety
- Feeling tired or yawning excessively after a meal
- Bloating in the gut, feeling nauseous, excessive belching, diarrhea, loose stools
- Unexplained muscle and joint pain

ALLERGY
SYMPTOMS

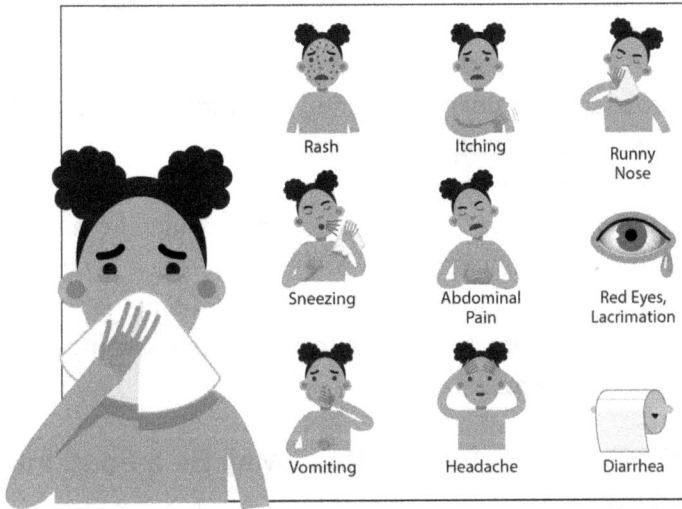

ALLERGY
TRIGGERS

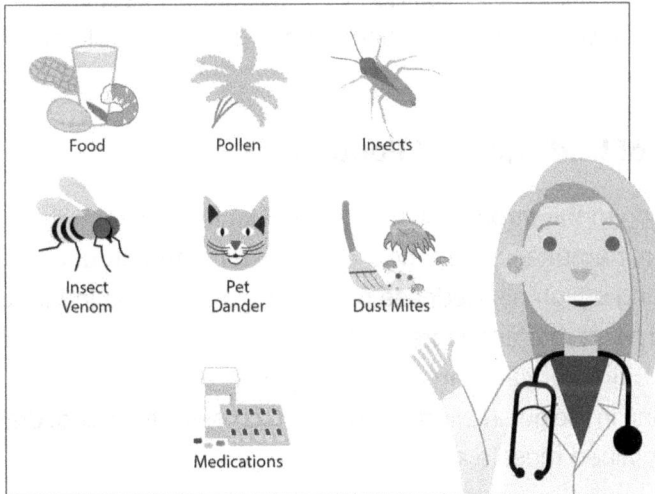

Figure 2: Symptoms and triggers of allergy.

Reactions Can Be Triggered by a Range of Substances

While this book is primarily concerned with reactions to food, it's important to understand that insect bites, latex, drugs, pollen, and other substances can also trigger reactions, some of which can be life-threatening.

Many Reactions Have Look-Alike Symptoms

Visible symptoms of reactions can range from mildly bothersome to life-threatening. For example, diarrhea, abdominal pain, and nausea can signal food intolerance (such as lactose intolerance) or a food allergy. However, if those symptoms escalate to swelling of the throat and breathing problems, a severe food allergy may be in play and anaphylaxis may be the result.

Since both allergies and intolerances can cause nausea and digestive distress after eating, what's the difference? Whereas an upset stomach from a food intolerance will be over after the food has passed through the digestive system, a true allergic reaction to a food could escalate into a serious medical emergency. No, not all food allergies are severe, but the potential exists for increasing severity over time and escalating symptoms during a reaction.

What You Might Think Is a Food Allergy May Be a Food Intolerance

About 26 million (11%) of American adults have been diagnosed with a food allergy. Around 19% of U.S. adults *believe* they are allergic to certain foods when it's more likely they have a food intolerance (Gupta 2019). After years of observing and treating patients, I believe these statistics do not adequately reflect the great number of people who suffer for years from undiagnosed allergies *and* intolerances, simply because they don't know help is available.

Symptoms of Undiagnosed Food Allergies:

- Swelling in the throat, which can feel like having something stuck there
- Itching, numbness, and tingling on the face and around the mouth
- A feeling of lightheadedness caused by a decrease in blood pressure
- Rapid heart rate and increased anxiety
- Feeling tired or yawning excessively after a meal
- Bloating in the gut, feeling nauseous, excessive belching, diarrhea, loose stools
- Unexplained muscle and joint pain

LACTOSE INTOLERANCE
SYMPTOMS

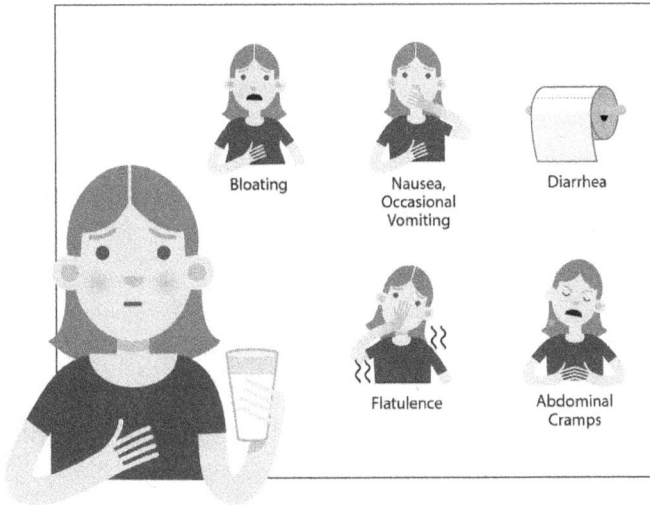

Bloating

Nausea,
Occasional
Vomiting

Diarrhea

Flatulence

Abdominal
Cramps

LACTOSE INTOLERANCE
MANAGEMENT

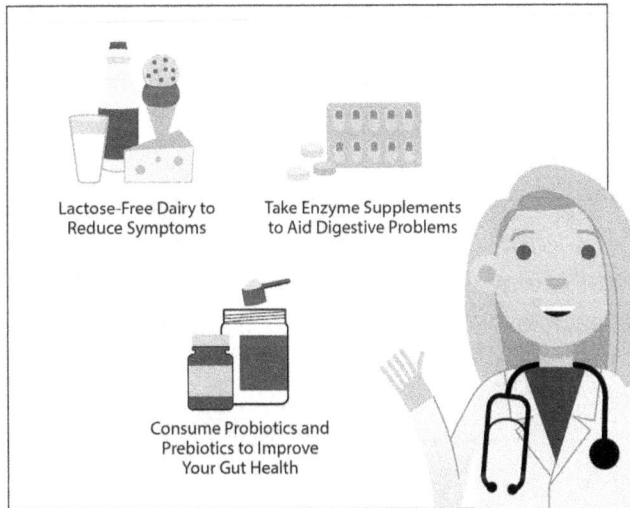

Lactose-Free Dairy to
Reduce Symptoms

Take Enzyme Supplements
to Aid Digestive Problems

Consume Probiotics and
Prebiotics to Improve
Your Gut Health

Figure 3: Symptoms and management strategies for lactose intolerance.

What Is a Food Allergy vs. a Food Intolerance?

Children with a food allergy have immune systems that react to certain proteins found in food. In most instances, a food allergy comes on suddenly and can be triggered by even just a small amount of food.

A food intolerance does not involve the immune system; therefore, symptoms are generally less severe than those from a food allergy. Digestive problems are common complaints associated with a food intolerance, such as lactose intolerance.

Examples of reactions that are quite real but are not caused by allergy to food include:

1. Allergic reaction to medications or other substances that happen to occur at the time of ingestion
2. Metabolic issues (lactose intolerance)
3. Toxic reaction (food poisoning)
4. Chemical effects (rhinitis from hot/spicy foods)
5. Gustatory flushing (flushing while eating)
6. Pharmacologic reactions (typically to substances like alcohol or caffeine)
7. Irritant reactions (in patients with irritant-type contact allergy and especially those with atopic dermatitis)
8. Infections
9. Idiosyncratic (unexplained) reactions, such as those to sulfites, nitrites, or MSG

Allergic Reactions Involve One or More Body Systems

Symptoms of a mild allergic reaction affect one organ system. For example, hay fever affects the upper respiratory system. Non-allergic reactions like food intolerance generally affect one primary body system, too. For example, symptoms of lactose intolerance affect the gastrointestinal system with bloating, nausea, etc. In contrast, a severe allergic reaction involves two or more body systems.

Below, the World Allergy Organization Reaction Grading System details the primary symptoms at each level of allergic reaction.

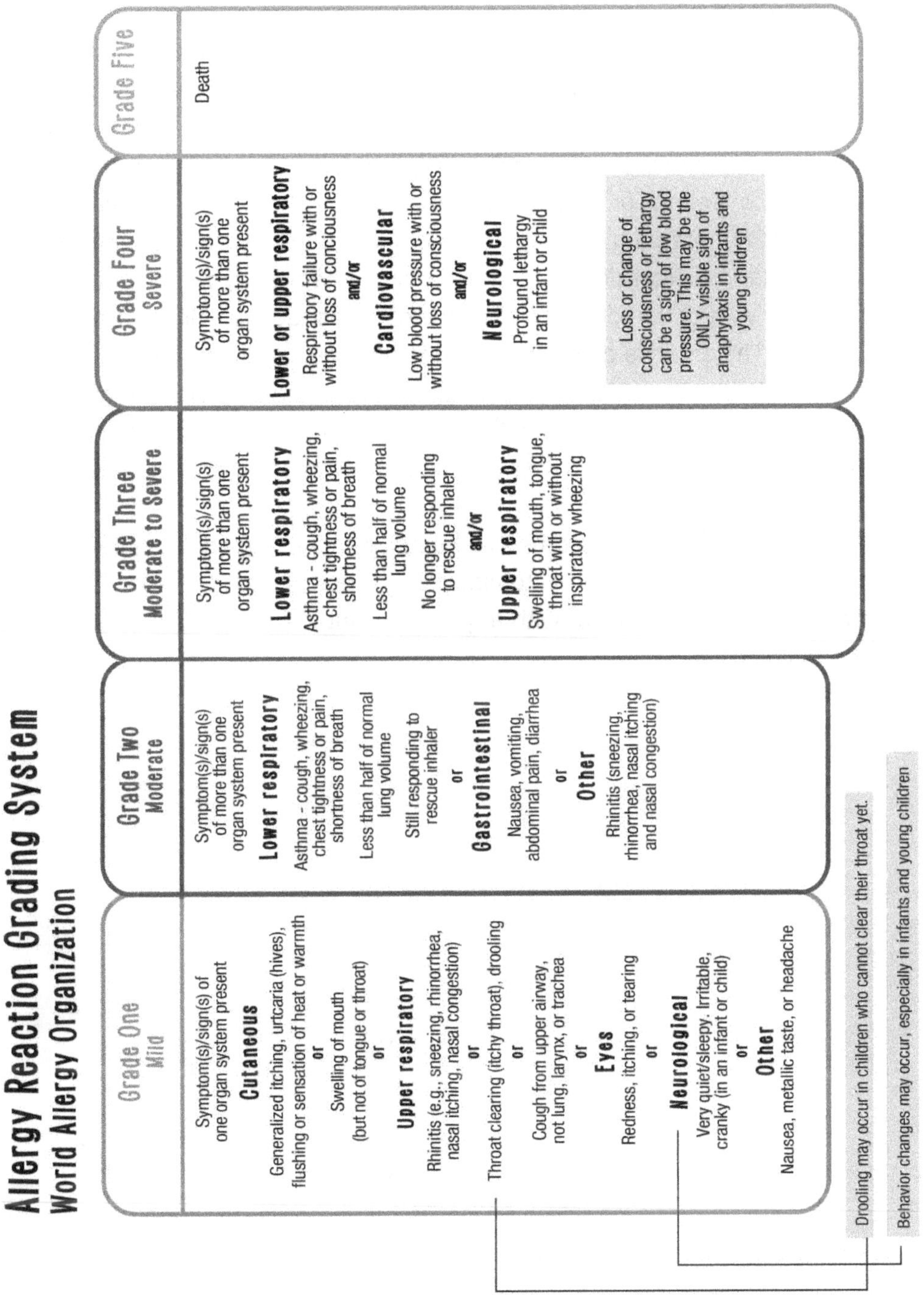

Allergy Reaction Grading System
World Allergy Organization

Grade One Mild	Grade Two Moderate	Grade Three Moderate to Severe	Grade Four Severe	Grade Five
Symptom(s)/sign(s) of one organ system present	Symptom(s)/sign(s) of more than one organ system present	Symptom(s)/sign(s) of more than one organ system present	Symptom(s)/sign(s) of more than one organ system present	Death
Cutaneous Generalized itching, urticaria (hives), flushing or sensation of heat or warmth *or* Swelling of mouth (but not of tongue or throat) *or*	**Lower respiratory** Asthma - cough, wheezing, chest tightness or pain, shortness of breath Less than half of normal lung volume Still responding to rescue inhaler *or*	**Lower respiratory** Asthma - cough, wheezing, chest tightness or pain, shortness of breath Less than half of normal lung volume No longer responding to rescue inhaler *and/or*	**Lower or upper respiratory** Respiratory failure with or without loss of conciousness *and/or*	
Upper respiratory Rhinitis (e.g., sneezing, rhinorrhea, nasal itching, nasal congestion) *or* Throat clearing (itchy throat), drooling *or*	**Gastrointestinal** Nausea, vomiting, abdominal pain, diarrhea *or* **Other** Rhinitis (sneezing, rhinorrhea, nasal itching and nasal congestion)	**Upper respiratory** Swelling of mouth, tongue, throat with or without inspiratory wheezing	**Cardiovascular** Low blood pressure with or without loss of consciousness *and/or*	
Cough from upper airway, not lung, larynx, or trachea *or* **Eyes** Redness, itching, or tearing *or*			**Neurological** Profound lethargy in an infant or child	
Neurological Very quiet/sleepy, Irritable, cranky (in an infant or child) *or* **Other** Nausea, metallic taste, or headache			Loss or change of consciousness or lethargy can be a sign of low blood pressure. This may be the ONLY visible sign of anaphylaxis in infants and young children	

Drooling may occur in children who cannot clear their throat yet.

Behavior changes may occur, especially in infants and young children

Figure 4: In this Allergy Reaction Grading System chart, The World Health Organization categorizes the symptoms of allergic reactions from mild to severe.

Notes to Figure 4:

i. Each grade is based on the organ system involved and severity. Organ systems are defined as: cutaneous, conjunctival, upper respiratory, lower respiratory, gastrointestinal, cardiovascular, and other. A reaction from a single organ system such as cutaneous, conjunctival, or upper respiratory, but not asthma, gastrointestinal, or cardiovascular is classified as a Grade 1. Symptom(s)/sign(s) from more than one organ system or asthma, gastrointestinal, or cardiovascular are classified as Grades 2 or 3. Respiratory failure or low blood pressure, with or without loss of consciousness, defines Grade 4 and death Grade 5. The grade is determined by the physician's clinical judgment.

ii. This constellation of symptoms may rapidly progress to a more severe reaction.

iii. Symptoms occurring within the first minutes after the injection may be a sign of severe anaphylaxis. Mild symptoms may progress rapidly to severe anaphylaxis and death.

iv. Sometimes signs or symptoms that occur are not included in the table, or the differentiation between a systemic reaction and vasovagal (vasodepressor) reaction, which may occur with any medical intervention, making differentiation difficult.

Chapter 2

Food Allergy Basics

Chapter Preview

- How do we develop food allergies?
- What is the most serious type of allergic reaction and what are the symptoms?
- What are the most common food allergens?

How Food Allergies Develop

Now that you are more familiar with reactions in general and the differences between allergic reactions, non-allergic reactions, and intolerances, this chapter will explore allergic reactions caused by foods.

A **food allergy** occurs when the body's immune system mistakenly perceives a certain food as harmful and reacts by causing one or more symptoms. This is called an **allergic reaction**. The food component that causes the allergic reaction (usually a protein) is called the allergen.

Your immune system's job is to protect your body from infection, parasites, certain molds, and viruses. In people who have allergies, the immune system attacks benign substances as if they were dangerous invaders. For example, the peanut cells pictured are harmless to most people. But because the allergic person's immune system has misidentified peanut as dangerous, it attacks the pollen with the histamines that cause allergic symptoms such as a runny nose.

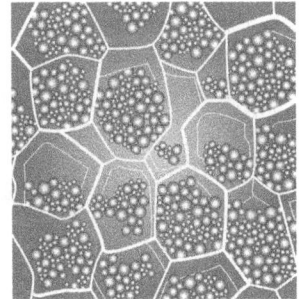

Figure 5: Scanning electron micrograph of peanut.

This drawing just looks like something from a foreign planet, maybe even something dangerous, doesn't it? Well, on a *Honey, I Shrunk the Kids* level, your body reacts like it is, too, often unnecessarily, in that it fights these little peanut proteins. Really, if it was not for the body's overreaction during allergy or anaphylaxis, they would be harmless.

Three Types of Reactions, Two Types of Allergies

There are two different types of allergic reactions, and a third type of reaction called a food intolerance, which is not an allergy but, rather, a definite medical condition in response to a food.

1. **Allergy - Immunoglobulin E (IgE)-mediated**. Symptoms result from the body's immune system making Immunoglobulin E (IgE) antibodies. These IgE antibodies react with specific foods.

2. **Allergy - Non IgE-mediated.** Other parts of the body's immune system react to a certain food. This reaction causes symptoms but does not involve an IgE antibody. Someone can have both IgE-mediated and non IgE-mediated food allergies.

3. **Not an Allergy - Food Intolerances.** Can be caused by the inability to properly digest a food and the resulting symptoms, a side effect (like a drug) of a food that was digested, or a chemical response to the food.

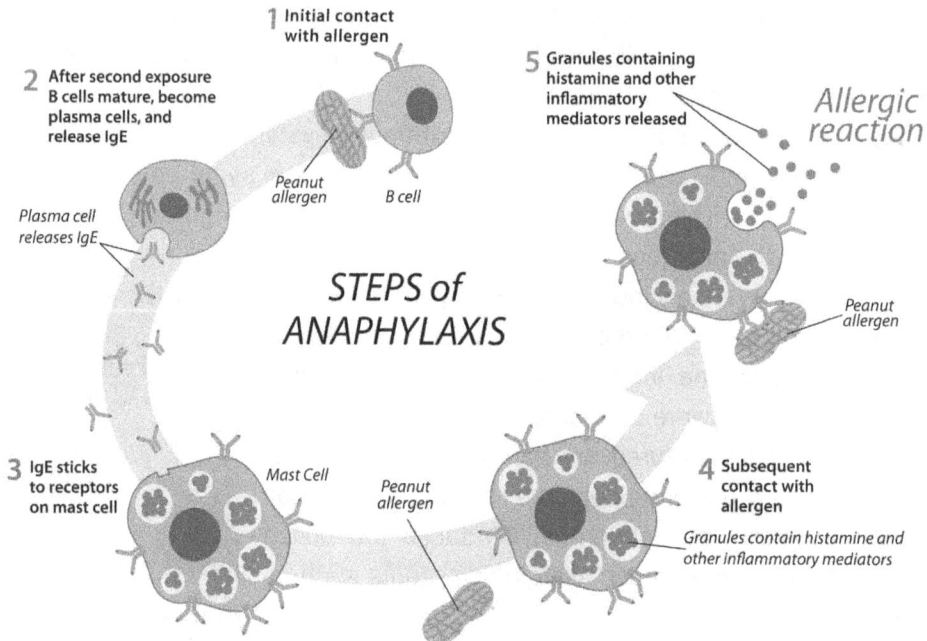

Figure 6: Steps of Anaphylaxis.

Notes to Figure 6:

When a food protein—in this case, peanut—meets a B cell for the first time, the peanut protein attaches to the B cell receptor on its surface where the B cell can interact with other cells in the environment of allergic cytokines. This exposure creates the initial sensitization. The B cells mature to plasma cells and the type of immune response—in this case, allergy—is locked in. On second exposure, better, more specific, and more tightly-binding antibodies are formed by the B cells. Because the B cell was exposed to allergic cytokines, they now create IgE, the allergic flag. Because the B cell is matured to a plasma cell, these IgE are released into circulation. After second exposure, the resulting peanut-specific IgE antibodies stick to the receptor sites on mast cells. When two or more IgEs are cross-linked, it causes the cell to be excited, releasing the mediators of allergy, including histamine, and creating all the symptoms of an allergic response.

How Does Immediate Food Allergy Occur?

When allergenic foods are eaten, they are broken down in the digestive tract, creating antigens (the allergic segment of food), which are absorbed. To the immune system, the allergic proteins create patterns that look very much like parasites, which cause the immune system to respond defensively. However, since food and pollen are benign, this overreaction is known as an allergy or hypersensitivity. What makes food and other allergens look like parasites to the immune system? On a microscopic level, it is the multiple repeating patterns that trigger the alarm.

Food allergy requires two exposures to an allergen to lock in an allergic response. The first exposure to the allergen sensitizes the immune system and sets the tone for the immune response.

This two-stage sensitization is like a biological war game (see fig. 6). When a food protein (in the case of a food allergy) meets a B cell for the first time and is recognized, the B cell receptor carries the food protein to its surface, where the B cell and the food protein can interact with other cells that set the stage for an allergic reaction by flooding the local environment with allergic cytokines, which are like hormones of the immune system.

This first exposure creates the initial sensitization. It is at this stage that those B-cells with B-cell receptors that can effectively latch onto the food protein and then divide and multiply, while those that do not die off. Also, it is at this stage that the type of allergic response is set. If this reaction occurs in an environment with cytokines that create an allergic response, then future responses to the food protein will be allergic.

On second exposure, better, more specific, and more tightly binding antibodies are formed by the B cells. Because the B cell was previously exposed to allergic-type cytokines, it now creates IgE (the allergic flag) and, because the B cell matures to a plasma cell, these IgE are released into circulation. This two-exposure process is why allergist-immunologists ask about previous exposures.

After the second exposure, the resulting IgE antibodies specific to the food allergen stick to the receptor sites on mast cells. Mast cells are the master allergic cells that release histamine and other mediators that promote allergic reactions (sneezing, wheezing, flushing, hives, etc.) and inflammation. When two or more IgE are cross-linked (meaning they are held together in close proximity by a single allergen), it causes the mast cell to be excited and to release the chemical mediators of allergy, creating all the symptoms of an allergic response.

antibody = immunoglobulin = immune system flags

There are four types of immunoglobulin: A, G, M, and E. IgE = allergic flag

IgE antibodies normally target parasites, as opposed to other foreign invaders, but IgE antibodies are formed under pressure from allergic hormones known as cytokines.

IgE is also responsible for recognizing allergens and causing allergic reactions, which is why I call them allergic flags.

Table 1

Entry Points for Allergens/Routes of Acquisition		
Route	**Main Organ Affected**	**Typical Allergens**
Inhalation, breathing in	Lungs, airway	Pollens, house dust, animal dander, latex
Contact with mucous membranes	Nose and eyes	Pollen
1. Skin contact 2. Ingestion, various	Skin	1. Various foods, uncertain 2. Drugs/medication
Ingestion, swallowed	Intestinal tract	Various foods, medication
All of the above	Systemic (whole body)	1. Insect venom 2. Drugs/medication 3. Foods

Main Symptoms	Disease
Wheezing, shortness of breath, fast and shallow breathing	Asthma
Runny nose, red, itchy, watery eyes	Hay fever, pink eye, rhinitis (common cold symptoms)
1. Itchy blisters 2. Large, itchy, fluid-filled blisters	1. Eczema 2. Hives
Vomiting, diarrhea	Allergic gastroenteropathy
Shock, sudden drop in blood pressure, wheezing	Anaphylaxis

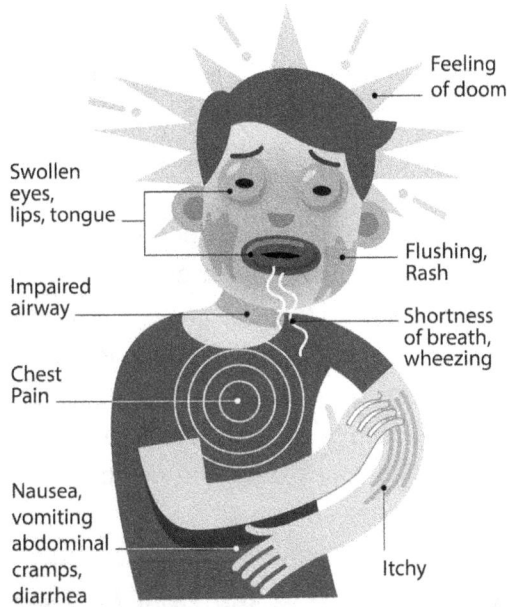

Swollen
eyes,
lips, tongue

Impaired
airway

Chest
Pain

Nausea,
vomiting
abdominal
cramps,
diarrhea

Feeling
of doom

Flushing,
Rash

Shortness
of breath,
wheezing

Itchy

Figure 7: Severe symptoms of anaphylaxis.

What is Immediate Food Allergy? Anaphylactic Response

The most concerning allergic reaction to food is immediate (or Type I) allergy and is known as *anaphylaxis*. This is a horrible-sounding word for a horrible process—the child's entire body reacts violently in response to a food, many times surprising the parents (see Chapter 6 for important details about anaphylaxis).

What Are the Symptoms of Immediate Food Allergy?

Examples of Immediate Food Allergy

Immediate food allergy is generally defined as a condition in which patients develop symptoms due to an allergic reaction to food within an immediate period, typically around 60 minutes (and frequently much sooner) after intake of causative foods. Some food allergy reactions are milder, like allergic rhinitis. Other food allergy reactions can be very severe, even life-threatening, like anaphylaxis, angioedema, and asthma. These reactions, by definition, typically happen very quickly after ingestion of the food allergen. These life-threatening allergic reactions are some of the scariest I treat for both patients and their families; I worry about each patient until I know they're going to be all right.

Mild symptoms of immediate food allergy include everything from sneezing and a runny nose to itchy, red, runny eyes.

Severe symptoms of immediate food allergy can include shortness of breath, wheezing, hoarseness, nausea, abdominal pain, diarrhea, vomiting, hives, itching, flushing, low blood pressure, cramping and loss of bladder and bowel control, and can lead to loss of consciousness and death.

Prevention of death by anaphylaxis involves countering and controlling any symptom that will cause death. This includes using epinephrine, first and foremost, because it acts quickly to counteract the most serious symptoms. As its name implies, it is the same as the "fight or flight" hormone and acts to increase blood pressure, open the airway, and arrest the remaining symptoms. It is critical that any child or adult with anaphylaxis has immediate access to an epinephrine auto-injector (pen) and knows how to use it or is being carefully monitored by a responsible adult while eating and snacking (see Chapter 6, Anaphylaxis).

Top Nine Most Common Food Allergens

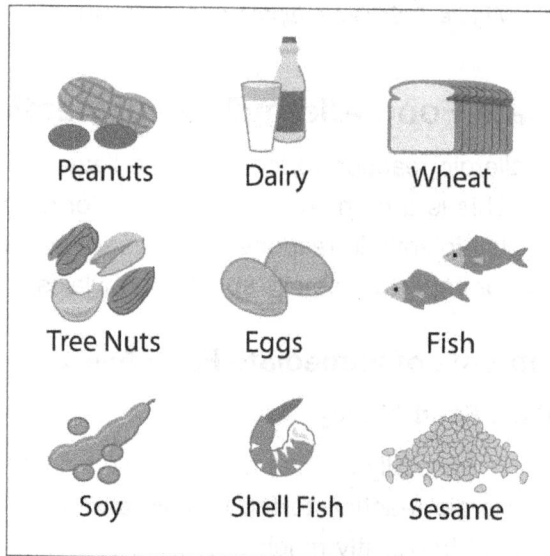

Figure 8: Most common food allergies.

Top Nine Food Allergies
Among 35 million allergy patients

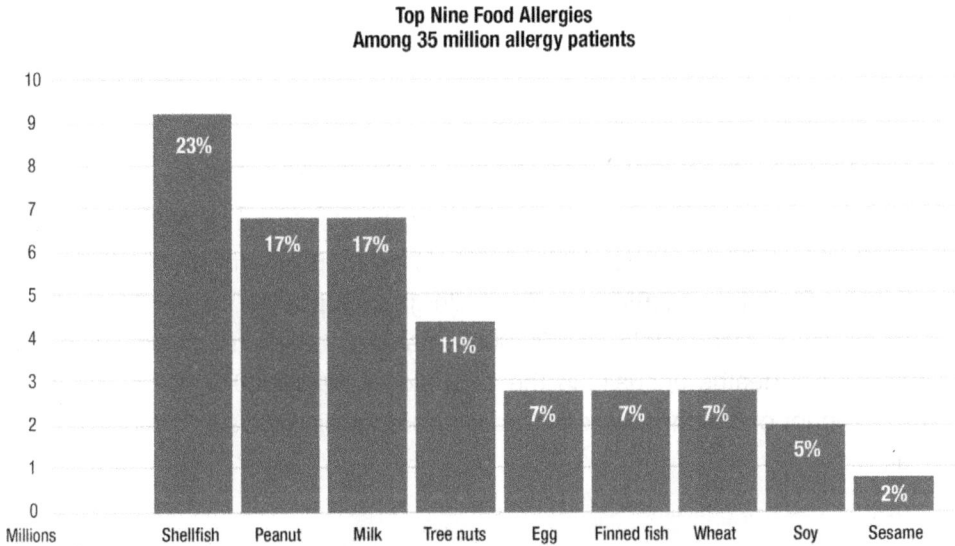

Figure 9: Over 35 million patients in the United States have allergies to these nine foods.

Examples of Common Food Allergens

The most common anaphylaxis triggers in children are food allergies, such as allergies to peanuts and tree nuts, egg, fish, shellfish, wheat, soy, sesame, and milk.

Although not common, some people develop anaphylaxis from aerobic exercise, such as jogging, or even less intense physical activity, such as walking. Eating certain foods before exercise and exercising when the weather is hot, cold, or humid also have been linked to anaphylaxis in some of these people.

Rapid changes in outside air temperature from warm to moderate to cold and changes in humidity can also increase the likelihood of anaphylaxis. Every year around Halloween, I see an increase in flares due to children being outside in the middle of the changing seasons.

Besides allergy to peanut, egg, tree nuts, fish, sesame, and shellfish, anaphylaxis triggers include:

- Medications, including antibiotics, aspirin, and other pain relievers available with or without a prescription, and the intravenous (IV) contrast used in some imaging tests
- Stings from bees, yellow jackets, wasps, hornets, and fire ants
- Latex
- Animals
- Pollen and molds in the environment
- Vaccines
- Just about anything to which you can be exposed

The more active allergies your child has at a particular time, the more likely it is they will have an allergic reaction and the more likely the reaction will be of greater severity.

You are not alone – the widespread impact of childhood allergies

Of the estimated 32 million people that have food allergies in the United States (Gupta 2019, 2018), 26 million are adults (Gupta 2019) and 5.6 million are children (Gupta 2018). Of all U.S. children, 7.6% have food allergies (Gupta 2019).

Food allergy is responsible for 200,000 emergency department admissions per year and 60-200 deaths annually in the U.S. alone (Radke 2017) (CDC 2022). The significant impact of childhood allergies is why proper diagnosis and intervention are essential.

Part 2: Immediate-Type Allergy

Chapter 3

Testing for Food Allergies

Chapter Preview

- What are the most effective ways an allergist tests for food allergies?
- Why your patient history is essential for a correct diagnosis.
- Why the oral food challenge is the gold standard in allergy testing.
- Which unreliable testing methods you'll want to avoid.

Testing for Allergies Starts with a Thorough Patient History

Before we do any testing, we will discuss the patient's history in detail. That history will tell me—often quite clearly—to which food(s) and/or substances the patient is hypersensitive. The patient's history usually connects the dots between the exposure and the allergic reaction and, conversely, between no exposure and a lack of reaction. In addition, the patient's suspicion is sometimes (one of) the best clues we have in determining the trigger of their reaction. For immediate-type allergies, the story is usually cut and dried.

The patient's history will also enable me to establish a pre-test probability, a subjective but educated guess of the likelihood that there is an allergy and its cause. Testing then confirms my pre-test probability, although tests are not 100% accurate.

The immune system is an amazingly complex body system and, while allergy testing becomes more accurate and helpful every year, both skin and blood testing can yield false positives and false negatives. This is one of the reasons your allergist-immunologist's experience and judgment are essential for interpreting the testing along with your or your child's history.

Which Is Better – A Skin Test or Blood Test?

To maximize my accuracy and judgment of safety, I prefer to conduct both skin and blood testing. If a patient has had severe food reactions, I will start with blood testing because it will not cause an allergic reaction, which can happen with skin testing. However, if the blood test results are negative or equivocal, I will follow up with a skin test. If a patient has not had a severe reaction and I do not anticipate one, I will conduct both blood and skin testing.

Food-specific IgE blood testing may be costlier than skin prick tests and the number of foods that can be tested by blood can be limited. It may also take longer to obtain results.

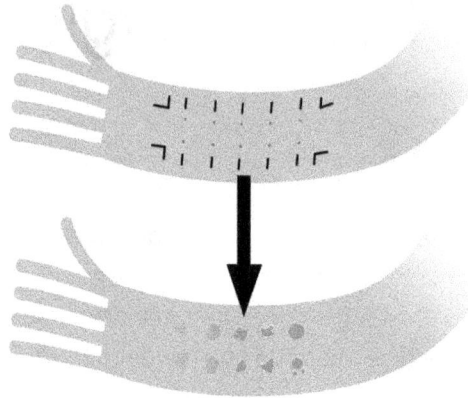

Figure 10: Example of the wheal and flare reaction from a skin prick test.

Skin Testing Is Highly Sensitive, Less Specific, and Test Results Are Available Same Day

Skin tests are methods of testing for allergic antibodies that are actually engaged on an allergic cell and in high enough concentration to create an allergic reaction. A skin test introduces small amounts of the suspected substance or allergen into the scratched skin and, after 20 minutes, the development of each reaction to the suspected allergen is recorded.

The scratching of the skin (also known as the prick method skin test) introduces the potential triggers into the epidermal layer just underneath the top of the skin (Cox 2008). This is the top layer of skin; it lies just above the dermal layer containing the master allergic cells, known as mast cells. If the mast cells have allergic flags or antibodies attached to their surface that recognize the trigger, once the trigger is introduced into the same layer, it can activate the mast cells, causing them to release histamine, leukotrienes, and other chemicals.

Histamine then causes leakage of the blood vessels of the skin, creating a little raised area known as a wheal, and dilation of the blood vessels of the skin, which creates an area of redness around the wheal, which is known as a flare. Together, the wheal and flare make up a hive. Therefore, skin testing is a controlled hive reaction. Only allergies that are recognized result in a hive under most circumstances. The hive is measured and interpreted by an allergist-immunologist.

This corresponds to the last step of the allergic reaction described in Chapter 2. In other words, the immune system has already been exposed to the allergen and has already committed to responding to that allergen with an allergic response.

Patients need to be off antihistamine medications for about seven days prior to skin testing so the antihistamine does not block histamine production and interrupt the wheal and flare reaction of the test.

Medical-grade skin tests for allergies
Test sensitivity, specificity, and error rate

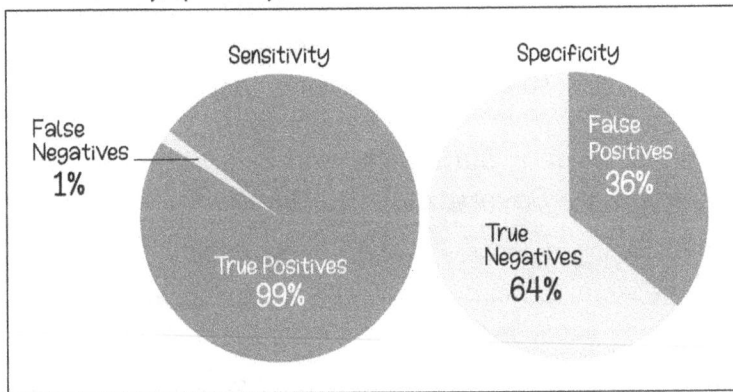

Figure 11: The diagnostic value of a food allergy skin test lies in the test's sensitivity and specificity.

How Effective Is Skin Testing for Food Allergy?

Allergist-immunologists are careful to choose medical-grade test instruments that are as accurate and reliable as possible and continually work to recognize their advantages and limitations, as well as how to effectively interpret the results.

The diagnostic value of a food allergy skin test lies in the test's sensitivity and specificity. The higher the degree of sensitivity and specificity, the more the test contributes to the doctor's analysis and diagnosis. The best available medical-grade skin tests we use generally have a high degree of **sensitivity** (very successful in detecting foods a patient is allergic to) and a lower degree **specificity** (less successful in detecting foods a patient is *not* allergic to). Knowing this, we expect test findings that include false positives and false negatives and take that into consideration when we choose a test instrument, understanding that it is more important to accurately detect food allergies than to rule out food allergies. This is one of the reasons we recommend testing only suspected foods rather than testing for a full panel. In circumstances where there is no idea which food(s) may be an issue or when there is food aversion, more extensive testing may be valuable.

The **sensitivity** of our skin tests is up to 99% successful in identifying the exact foods to which a patient is allergic. This is called a true positive result. The false negative error rate of these tests is very low; they fail to identify an existing food allergy only about 1% of the time. This test result is called a false negative because the patient's allergy to a specific food is not correctly detected.

The other measure of our tests' diagnostic value is **specificity**, the ability to ***rule out*** specific food allergies. Our tests will successfully identify about 64% of those foods to which the patient is *not* allergic and are safe for them to eat. This is a true negative result. The false positive error rate of these tests is higher. On average, this test **fails** to identify about 36% of those foods as safe for the patient to eat, giving a false positive result.

Understanding the limitations of these tests, the doctor will interpret the results and, with additional analysis and possibly more testing, determine which of those identified foods are, in fact, safe to eat and attempt to not limit the patient's diet.

Blood Testing Has Similar Sensitivity and Specificity to Skin Tests; Test Results May Take Several Days to Weeks

In contrast, blood testing measures how much specific IgE is in serum. In blood testing, the level of serum IgE can vary greatly and is highest about four weeks after exposure.

Blood testing is preferred if a patient cannot stop their antihistamines, has skin issues that would worsen on allergen exposure, if exposure would be dangerous and potentially cause an anaphylactic reaction, or if the stakes of being wrong are high. In these cases, testing both ways may be preferable.

Results of blood testing are delayed by processing time at a laboratory, typically from two to four weeks—at least, that is the general time frame for the labs in my clinic area.

In summary, if asked which is better, blood or skin testing, my answer is frequently both. However, it depends on the patient and the details of the allergic reaction.

Blood Testing for Food Allergies

Blood testing enables the patient to be tested without direct exposure to the allergen, which increases patient safety in cases of severe allergy or severe eczema (when the skin is not intact).

In blood testing, the patient's serum contains allergic antibodies (or IgE) that are exposed to multiple solid matrices embedded with the potential allergic triggers, e.g. one matrix for milk, one matrix for egg, etc.

If the patient's serum has IgE specific to these triggers, the trigger-specific IgE will stick to the matrix containing it. For example, if the patient is allergic to milk but not to egg, they will have milk-specific IgE, but no IgE that recognizes egg. Thus, IgE from this patient will attach to the solid matrix attached to milk proteins but not to the one with egg proteins attached (see fig. 12). The matrix with milk protein will register as positive and that with egg will register negative.

To increase the specificity of the blood testing results, a second antibody targeted to IgE is added. This second antibody has a measurable label such as a radioactive label or a fluorescent label. After a proper incubation, any excess antibody is rinsed away and the label is counted. The count (of radioactivity or level of fluorescence) is proportional to the amount of anti-milk IgE in this example. There are various ways of doing this, but this is the general method.

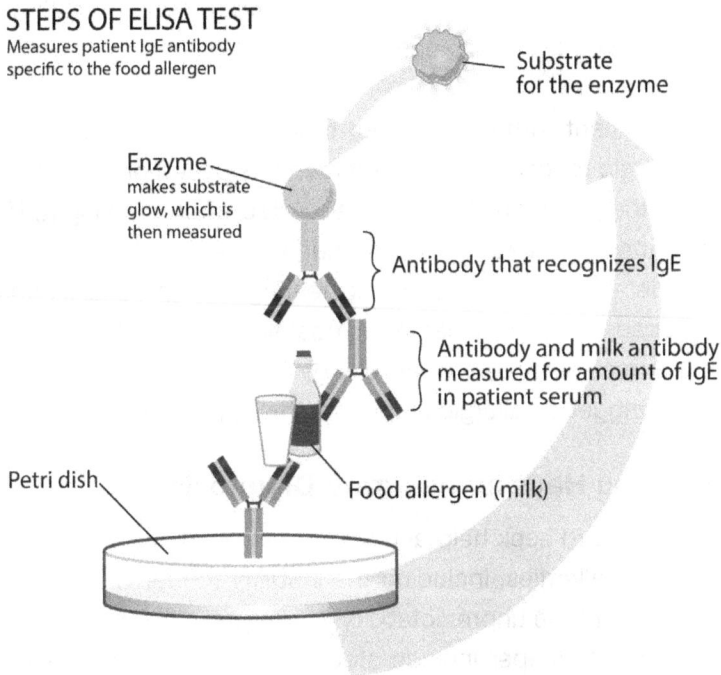

STEPS OF ELISA TEST
Measures patient IgE antibody
specific to the food allergen

Substrate
for the enzyme

Enzyme
makes substrate
glow, which is
then measured

Antibody that recognizes IgE

Antibody and milk antibody
measured for amount of IgE
in patient serum

Petri dish

Food allergen (milk)

Figure 12: Above is an illustration of one of these food allergy tests.

What If All Test Results Are Negative?

There are several reasons why the test results might be negative:

- Test gave a false negative due to the allergic chemical cascade present immediately after a reaction;
- Incorrect assumption about which allergen was the trigger;
- Misidentifying the reaction as allergic when it was not;

- It is an "idiopathic anaphylaxis," which means we have ruled out everything we can think of; or
- The reaction was due to a food intolerance, food aversion, or a side-effect of a drug or toxin.

When the test is negative, it is typically repeated in 3-6 months.

There Is No Perfect Test

If your child has a serious allergy, he/she really should see a board-certified allergist-immunologist because they are experts at interpreting allergy tests. Now, some allergists' approach is to prove an allergy with testing to avoid "wasting money." My approach is the opposite. I first eliminate concerns about foods to which the patient is not truly allergic.

If I challenge a patient with a suspected food, I am 99% certain they can safely eat it without an allergic reaction. My near-certainty is based on the pre-test possibility I surmised from the patient history and calculated after studying it. If the pre-test probability is high, the estimated results are much better.

Another consideration when interpreting testing is that sensitization can occur *without* allergy. Because the body has an almost limitless ability to make IgE, a test may cause an incorrect diagnosis of an allergy because of excess IgE or IgE that would not normally trigger an allergic response; this is known as a false positive.

Don't Quit Until You Have an Accurate Diagnosis

There are many reasons to seek help and support in pursuing an accurate diagnosis and treatment plan for allergies, including the inability to identify the allergy, inability to avoid the allergen, and the unpredictability of allergenic symptoms.

Other reasons to dig deeper include stools that are bleeding, black, or bloody; lack of appetite and early satiety; significant and unintentional weight loss; symptoms that awaken your child from sleep; sudden and significantly increased symptom severity; presence of iron-deficiency anemia or another form of malnutrition; and increased frequency of infections.

Some medical illnesses affect the way the body metabolizes and processes food. These include but are not limited to issues such as thyroid disease, diabetes, vitamin deficiency, and anemia. Ruling them out may be part of the initial diagnostic process by the pediatrician and specialists.

Certain family history should also trigger pursuit of another diagnosis or may require more help. Family medical histories of particular concern include inflammatory bowel syndrome (Crohn's disease or ulcerative colitis), celiac disease, colon cancer, rheumatologic disease, blood vessel abnormalities like vasculitis or aneurysms, and any syndromic or genetic disease. These and any other significant and life-changing diagnosis in a family member should always be mentioned to every physician.

Fasting and Refeeding Is a Method of Clarifying Positive Test Results

If the skin or blood test is positive but the reaction *is clearly not anaphylactic* or if the patient requests a full food allergy panel and the results show many positive reactions, the allergist-immunologist may request a limited time trial of fasting and refeeding each of the suspected foods. Any foods that do not result in allergic symptoms can then be added back to the diet.

As an allergist-immunologist, I conduct fasting and refeeding most typically with adults. For those who believe their hives are connected to a food allergy, I often try to identify safe foods they can eat while they are fasting and refeeding to discover the real source of their hives. My tactic is an attempt to prevent food aversions.

Children have much higher nutritional requirements to support their growth. If I think a parent is avoiding a particular food that is not likely to be an allergy, I may perform an oral food challenge to prove it.

Oral Food Challenge – The Gold Standard in Diagnosing Allergies

The oral food challenge (OFC) is a highly accurate diagnostic test for food allergies and is considered the gold standard. When an allergist-immunologist follows the thorough guidelines and standards developed by the medical community, studies have shown OFCs to be safe. Indeed, thousands have been performed worldwide with an excellent safety record. Additional benefits of an oral food challenge are as follows:

1. Safety – There is a risk of conducting an oral food challenge: a severe and potentially life-threatening allergic reaction can occur. In that case, the allergist-immunologist is literally at the patient's side and able to administer the appropriate medical help. Safety is the most important reason the allergist-immunologist conducts the food challenge in their clinic and oversees the entire process.
2. Precise Test Administration – An oral food challenge is conducted in the allergist-immunologist's office to ensure proper administration, precise dosing, and adherence to necessary wait times.
3. Real-Time Observation and Test Results – The allergist-immunologist provides constant, close observation of the patient's reaction to the implicated food and identifies his/her tolerance of increased doses and the maximum quantities tolerated.
4. Comprehensive Diagnosis – The allergist-immunologist is best equipped to

reach a diagnosis when the results of the oral food challenge are considered along with the patient's history and other test results.

5. Clarity – Knowing exactly which foods you can and cannot eat will reduce your anxiety about everything from grocery shopping to meal preparation to meals away from home. An oral food challenge provides that level of clarity for each food tested. In the best circumstances, the patient's diet can be expanded—sometimes greatly—and vigilance in shopping for and preparing food can be relaxed.

Preparation for an Oral Food Challenge

The best preparation for an oral food challenge is being healthy; being ill or dehydrated could increase the risk of reaction or make resuscitation more challenging in case of an allergic reaction. All chronic conditions, like asthma, should be under control. The allergist-immunologist will give advance instructions about medications (e.g. antihistamines are typically stopped one week prior to the oral food challenge).

Sometimes, the patient's parent(s) will be recruited to prepare the food for the oral food challenge, usually with a recipe and guidance provided by the allergist-immunologist. In these cases, it is important to follow the recipe exactly so the amount of allergenic protein ingested is known. This may be necessary based on which foods are stocked in the allergy lab, the level of preparation required, and the pickiness or age of the child.

The Oral Food Challenge Process

Prior to the first day of the oral food challenge, the patient's vital signs are checked and a breathing test given to confirm they are in good health.

Next, the allergist-immunologist feeds small, carefully measured amounts of the suspected food to the patient followed by 15 to 30 minutes of close observation for any symptoms. If no reaction occurs, a slightly larger amount of the food is fed to the patient followed by another observation period. Any reaction that is concerning ends the challenge.

The final step of the oral food challenge is a prolonged observation period for the safety of the patient.

If a normal portion of the suspected food can be consumed without reaction, the test is regarded as negative and the food can be added back to the diet. On the other hand, if allergic symptoms occur, the reaction is considered positive, the test is aborted, and the food removed from the patient's diet.

Limitations of the Oral Food Challenge

An oral food challenge is a medical test used when a food is suspected of causing the patient an allergic reaction and will either confirm or rule out allergy. However, an oral food challenge may not provide adequate information for delayed allergies such as celiac disease and eczema, adverse effects of food, such as histamine toxicity, or anxiety from a traumatic experience with food. An alternate test may be more helpful for those types of allergies and conditions.

Sometimes, people confuse the oral food challenge with food oral immunotherapy. An oral food challenge is used to rule out (or validate) an anaphylactic reaction to a food, while food oral immunotherapy is therapy to increase the patient's tolerance of a food allergen with the intent that accidental ingestion at minimum and, ideally, liberal consumption may occur at some point without an allergic reaction or at least a survivable reaction (see Chapter 4).

Reversed Allergy Diagnosis

One successful oral food challenge made it possible for me to reverse a child's diagnosis of a fish allergy. In this case, fish had triggered a one-time anaphylactic reaction. I discovered it was not a true allergy, but scombroid (or histamine) poisoning. Happily, this child is eating fish regularly to this day.

While an oral food challenge should only be performed with the help and guidance of an allergist-immunologist, there is a great chance that infants and children at high risk of developing a food allergy can get help mitigating their risk.

Invalidated and Unproven Tests and Treatments

Many patients have been saddled with a label that they have a food allergy when it does not actually exist, due to improper interpretation of testing or invalid testing methods. In addition, they may have either been tested with non-IgE type tests or the tests were not interpreted with the limits of the test in mind.

While some of the following tests may eventually demonstrate usefulness, they have not been evaluated thoroughly enough for board-certified allergist-immunologists, including me, to be comfortable recommending them to other allergist-immunologists or my patients.

Testing Food-Specific IgG or Testing Specifically for IgG4

These tests have not been validated and do not have established sensitivity or specificity for detecting food allergy. In fact, high IgG4 is more likely to represent tolerance to a food or at least represent exposure. Further increase of food-specific IgG4 after completion of treatment with food oral immunotherapy seems to support this.

While there are some retrospective studies that support some relationship of food-specific IgG with inflammatory bowel syndrome symptoms, this has yet to be validated and accepted. However, it is established and well known that IgG antibodies are found in healthy patients (deficiency of IgG antibodies is treated as a primary immune disorder) and are more likely to be an indication of food intolerance than an allergy or inflammation (Kelso 2018). Currently, the American College of Allergy, Asthma, & Immunology and the American Academy of Allergy, Asthma, & Immunology do not recommend IgG or IgG4 subclass testing for foods.

Provocation-Neutralization Testing

Provocation-neutralization testing claims to identify food sensitivity by intradermal injection of foods (Kelso 2018). Provocation of the food-specific symptoms is interpreted as a positive test. The "neutralizing" dose is then re-administered to prevent symptoms when the patient eats that food. Studies of this technique show no difference between neutralization of the injected food and injection of the saline negative control. In other words, there is no scientific validity to this test.

Hair Analysis

A study of hair analysis samples sent hair from nonallergic subjects to three different labs, all of which resulted in positive and disparate results. This lack of reproducibility led the authors to suspect that this method could not be trusted (Kelso 2018; Sethi 1987).

ALCAT Test

The ALCAT test involves incubating the patient's white blood cells with foods that are potential triggers. The change in cell size that occurs both before and after this incubation is measured. A change of >13% is considered positive; a change of 9-13% is considered equivocal; and a change <9% is reported as negative. This information is used to generate a diet to alleviate a diverse group of symptoms and disorders. There are no studies in peer-reviewed literature that currently validate this test or its use in prescribing diet or treatment (Kelso 2018).

Electrodermal Testing

Electrodermal testing uses electrodes to measure the electric circuit between the electrodes when a small voltage is initiated through the circuit. Vials containing the suspected food are then included in the circuit. Impedance of the skin, which is like resistance but also includes the phase of the electric current, is then measured. This information is used to assess food sensitivity and to make decisions on re-challenging with the allergenic foods (Kelso 2018). There is no evidence to validate this testing for evaluating food allergy.

Applied Kinesiology/Muscle Testing

Food intolerance tested with applied kinesiology involves having the patient hold a vial of the test food while extending their opposite arm. A practitioner tries to depress the extended arm while the patient resists (Kelso 2018). Being able to depress the arm is a sign of weakness and interpreted as a sensitivity to the test food. There has not been sufficient peer-reviewed evidence to advocate for this testing as a reliable means of diagnosing allergy.

Summary of Findings of Invalidated Tests

If you are the parent of an allergic child, there are several dangers in trusting these testing methods and results. First, if a parent is told their child is not allergic to a food after using one of the above unreliable testing methods, the child could actually be allergic and in danger if they ingest the allergic food. Second, if the parent is told incorrectly that their child is allergic to a particular food when they're not, and the allergic food is avoided unnecessarily, the child could become malnourished and some experts theorize that prolonged avoidance could actually result in development of a food allergy.

There may be occasions when the test results, even of these invalidated tests, seem to align with clinical symptoms, that is, when avoidance of a positive food causes symptoms to resolve. This may be due to a true food intolerance. The foods that cause intolerance are widely known, so guessing is not challenging. A temporary elimination and reintroduction diet are typically all that is necessary to prove or disprove this information (see Chapter 20).

In summary, it is important to know that if you can mail-order a test or treatment, it's unlikely the test has been either reviewed or regulated by the FDA. While there may be reason to use non-FDA approved testing and treatment methods, that fact and the reason should be disclosed to the patient by the treating physician before testing.

Board-certified allergist-immunologists stay current on state-of-the art testing and treatment in the field, learn to read the literature, and interpret testing and treatment as sound, experimental, or unorthodox. There are never quick answers in medicine.

Chapter 4

Management Strategies for Severe Food Allergies

Chapter Preview

- What are the most effective management strategies for severe food allergies?
- What are the benefits and risks of those strategies?
- Why parents and the allergic child must be on constant alert for exposure to allergic triggers.

What Are the Best Management Strategies for Immediate Food Allergy?

There are two major approaches to the management of immediate (Type I) food allergy. The first is complete avoidance and the second is food immunotherapy.

Complete Avoidance of the Trigger Food Is the First Step to Preventing an Allergic Reaction

The fundamental decision every allergic person (and their family) must make is to avoid their allergens. From the moment of their diagnosis, every effort to eliminate those allergens from every part of their lives—home, school, brown-bag lunches, restaurant meals, meals at friends' homes—must be made. This is challenging, especially if the allergy is to one of the very common ingredients in food, such as milk, egg, and peanut.

Until recently, the first recommendation of the allergist-immunologist has been to avoid allergens to prevent anaphylaxis. However, it is difficult to strictly avoid common food allergens like milk and egg, because they are ingredients in many processed foods. Further, those same processed foods are laced with flavor- and texture-enhancing ingredients that may be allergens.

Also, we think this prolonged avoidance of foods, typically delayed until the child reaches 6 to 18 months of age, may actually *increase* the likelihood of food allergies. This is thought to be a result of removing the protection that regularly eating small amounts of potentially allergenic foods provides. Conversely, delaying this gradual increase in the allergens in the diet prevents this protection from occurring.

Parents, this means you must vigilantly read all food labels and exercise great caution in every situation where there is no control over food preparation such as in restaurants and in friends' homes. Further, you must ensure that everyone who interacts with your child is aware of their allergy and has all the information needed to quickly intervene should an accidental ingestion occur.

◆ ◆ ◆

As a mother of allergic children and an allergist-immunologist, I definitely live with and understand the significant challenges other allergy parents face. To highlight some of my own learning experiences, I will share a few stories. Telling them is a little embarrassing, but just like other allergy parents, it is very challenging for me to keep my own family's allergies, schedules, and schoolwork straight!

One of my child's best friends has a life-threatening peanut allergy, so I have always been very careful when he visits. Even so, when he and his mother arrived at my child's birthday party one year, his mother asked what we were serving. When I told her we were having little ice cream cups from a national food chain, she asked to see one. She looked at the package, turned the label over, and there it was in the ingredient list: peanut. I was so glad she never let her guard down! From then on, I was even more careful to read labels when her child was at our home.

This story shows how much I (and my colleagues) understand and appreciate the constant vigilance required from parents, family, and friends to protect a child with allergies. I sincerely hope those who don't have allergies or an allergic child appreciate the life-saving potential of the precautions parents take and don't perceive them as over-reactions.

A child with severe food allergies should be monitored by a responsible adult *every* time they eat, drink, or snack.

My second embarrassing story involves my oldest daughter, Katie. We were new at a peanut-free school—which meant that during snack time, no peanuts could be in any snack that might cause an issue for their peanut-allergic classmates. One morning, I asked my daughter to pack a snack for snack time. She did and I paid no attention because I never have to worry about Katie following instructions. Well, when she arrived home at the end of her school day, she told me her day had been terrible.

"Why?" I asked.

"Because I had to stand outside during snack!" Katie declared.

"Well, did you do something wrong?" I was surprised because Katie is my "perfect" child.

"No. My snack had peanuts in it," Katie said.

Oh, my goodness! Katie had packed a Kind bar for her snack (the first and quickest snack she could find) but when the teacher found out it contained peanuts, she was sent outside to eat it. (It is great that more and more teachers and school staff are looking out for their students in this way.)

My child's wonderful, peanut-free classroom was new even to me! I educated my daughter and it never happened again. The minor inconvenience of putting a bit more thought and effort into preparing a safe snack is nothing compared to the risk of exposing another child to a possible severe allergic reaction. And, with more and more allergic people, my children have more and more allergic friends who could be at risk.

The moral of these stories is: bring your own food and do not trust _anyone_ with your child's safety.

◆ ◆ ◆

Be Prepared for a Severe Reaction

Knowing that accidental exposure is likely to happen, especially for common allergies, I highly recommend that the patient carry an epinephrine pen, wear a medic alert bracelet or necklace, and carry an Anaphylaxis Action Plan to guide immediate treatment.

Beware of Cross-Contamination in Restaurants

Anyone with a food allergy knows cross-contamination can make dining out very risky because they must strictly avoid their food allergens. It is important to exercise caution in restaurants and on occasions when the patient and their family do not control preparation of the food. In particular, avoid restaurants where cross-contamination can easily occur. Cross-contamination happens when an allergenic food is mixed with or touches non-allergenic food, thereby making it unsafe for the highly allergic person to consume.

Restaurant workers, unless it is known that they have received significant education about food allergies, should not be considered knowledgeable about them; they are known to have common misconceptions about allergies (Radke 2017). For example, restaurant workers surveyed shared a common belief that the danger of food allergy would be avoided by picking the allergenic food out of the dish (Radke 2017). Any parent of an allergic child knows this is not true. The amount of food that can result in anaphylaxis is sometimes so minute, it is not at all visible. The concept that food allergy precautions are not more rigorously taught to "food preparers" blows my mind.

Be Aware of Cross-Reactive Foods

Further, the patient and family should be made aware of cross-reactive foods. Cross-reactive foods are those that an allergic person is more likely to react to because they have a common protein structure with the patient's allergenic food (see Oral Allergy Syndrome, Chapter 12).

Treatment with Food Oral Immunotherapy Increases Tolerance to the Allergen

Immunotherapy for allergies works by carefully exposing the patient's immune system to the allergen over time, thus building up tolerance and reducing the patient's risk of allergic reaction. Using your immune system as a barrier to allergens is the optimal solution for long-lasting results. The goal is to develop life-long immunity and to be free of medications.

The first type of immunotherapy most people think of are allergy shots. Over the years, allergist-immunologists have used allergy shots to stop or reduce patients' allergic reactions, especially for hay fever, pollen, etc. While there are no allergy shots for food allergies, sometimes, allergy shots for cross-reactive allergens can be variably helpful. Before food oral immunotherapy went "prime time," some allergists would use this to help reduce even slightly allergic reactions to food.

The most effective method of immunotherapy for Type I allergies is known as food immunotherapy. There are several approaches, but the basic idea is to start exposure at a quantity below the allergic threshold and increase it slowly, allowing regulatory cells to be produced that inhibit the allergic cells, thus lowering the risk of a reaction and, ideally, preventing future reactions.

Success in this area is defined as a majority of patients being able to accidentally ingest their allergen without anaphylaxis or, if they do have anaphylaxis, it is less severe. In some cases, the therapy is so successful that patients can freely eat their allergen.

Risks of FOIT

Food Oral Immunotherapy (FOIT) overall appears to be superior in terms of efficacy thus far. However, the side effect of anaphylaxis is lower in sublingual and patch immunotherapy.

There is now an FDA-approved Food Oral Immunotherapy capsule for peanut that has been in public use with considerable success. However, board-certified allergist-immunologists are not limited to what the FDA has approved as a drug. We give patients access to a broad range of foods for FOIT testing, which both simplifies the testing process and makes it less expensive. The FDA approval of these peanut capsules as treatment of peanut allergy has also caused many of us allergist-immunologists to scratch our heads: the FDA already oversees foods—how are they going to reclassify all the foods as drugs for the sake of Food Oral Immunotherapy (see Chapter 5)?

Therapy for Severe Food Allergies: Long-Term Relief is Achievable

Chapter Preview

- Can we prevent food allergies or reduce their severity?
- What is food oral immunotherapy?
- Learn how carefully controlled exposure to a food allergen can result in desensitization.

Food Oral Immunotherapy or Desensitization

Food oral immunotherapy (FOIT) is a carefully calibrated medical therapy that exposes the allergic person to their allergen for the purpose of desensitization or, said another way, to increase their tolerance threshold. **The life-changing results experienced by successful FOIT patients have given both parents and children new hope and inspiration.**

There are many benefits of food oral immunotherapy:

1. FOIT reduces the patient's risk of a severe reaction to their allergen(s).
2. At a minimum, FOIT seeks to reduce the intensity of an allergic reaction in the case of accidental ingestion.
3. The measure of successful food oral immunotherapy is if the patient will tolerate an accidental exposure to the allergen without having a severe reaction.

Food oral immunotherapy should be performed only by a board-certified allergist-immunologist (ABAI.org), as the risks can be serious. Because the actual food allergen is fed to the patient during FOIT, there is a risk of an allergic reaction, which could include hives, swelling, bronchospasm with difficulty breathing, loss of consciousness, and shock that may require emergency treatment and hospitalization. In rare cases, it can result in death.

The concept of food oral immunotherapy is not new. It was first attempted in

1908—the same year the term *allergy* was coined—by a physician named Alfred Schofield who desensitized a 13-year-old boy who was allergic to egg (Smith 2014).

The first FDA-approved form of immunotherapy is for those with peanut allergy, and utilizes a drug known as Palforzia (*arachis hypogaea* or peanut). This is intensely exciting, yet slightly confusing, because this is the first food that has been reclassified as a drug.

Laying the Groundwork for Successful FOIT

Food oral immunotherapy starts with a health evaluation of the allergic child and fine-tuning any disease states such as asthma and other allergies that might interfere with the FOIT process. Depending on the severity of symptoms, environmental allergen immunotherapy may be advised first. This is because FOIT may be going quite well but, due to the length of time it takes to accomplish tolerance, environmental allergies may start triggering other symptoms, worsen the symptoms from food, and/or increase the likelihood of an allergic reaction. To prevent interference of any kind during FOIT, it is best to address any other medical conditions ahead of time.

Overview of the FOIT Process

The first day of food oral immunotherapy is usually a half-day process, starting with ingestion of an amount of allergen below the allergenic threshold and feeding increasing amounts, unless symptoms necessitate stopping. Mild symptoms such as several hives, mild itching, or mild abdominal pain do not stop the therapy. However, severe or prolonged symptoms will necessitate stopping the process for safety. The final dose is followed by an extended period of observation, typically one hour.

After the clinic phase of the food oral immunotherapy is complete and the allergist-immunologist deems it safe to proceed, the follow-up home therapy phase begins. There, the desensitization process continues over a period of months with the patient taking the prescribed dose of the allergen each day. In the home therapy phase, no change in the dose amount or frequency should be attempted without specific instructions from the allergist-immunologist, due to the risk of anaphylaxis.

Precautions for the Home Phase of FOIT

Parents and caregivers are required to follow our FOIT rules and guidelines for safety reasons. If they cannot, it may not be the right time for you and your family to be in this therapeutic program. It is also a rather long process. If it cannot be undertaken start to finish, it probably should not be started. At the very least, its success should not be evaluated based on a half-hearted effort.

Home dosing is anxiety-provoking at first, but if you work closely with your allergist-immunologist, you can be successful. Following are some basic rules to lower the risk of a severe reaction and to prevent a reaction from culminating in a tragedy. Even though I'm providing a general overview of FOIT, all decisions to start, stop, or continue FOIT should be at the direction of the supervising allergist-immunologist.

- First and foremost, every parent needs to be aware of what to do in the uncommon but possible case of anaphylaxis. They must be capable of administering an epinephrine auto-injector to their child.
- The dose must *never* be escalated at home.
- If a dose is skipped for any reason, especially for illness, or if the instructions are not understood, call your allergist-immunologist's office for clarification and guidance.
- For at least one hour after each day's administration of the home dose, the child should not be permitted to fall asleep and should be observed.
- There should be no vigorous exercise for one hour before and two hours after administration of the food allergen.
- The same symptoms that apply to stopping a testing or challenge session also apply to initiating the Anaphylaxis Action Plan. That is, a mild reaction with a few hives, a little itch, or abdominal pain is reason to double-check that your arsenal of medications is nearby, but mild symptoms are not a reason to stop the therapy in general. If more severe symptoms appear, consult your allergist-immunologist.
- Stop FOIT if severe symptoms appear. Do not hesitate to give epinephrine as part of the patient's Anaphylaxis Action Plan.

Note: FOIT should never be given on an empty stomach, during an active gastrointestinal or other illness, or in a situation in which you could not get help for the child (like on a plane or just before boarding a plane).

Can Severe Food Allergies Be Prevented?

The idea of preventing food allergy started with the observation that children in countries that do not delay eating allergenic foods have a lower rate of allergy when compared with similar children in countries that avoid eating allergenic foods. In Israel, for example, Jewish children ages 8-14 months eat an average of about 7.1 grams of peanut protein each week and have a very low rate of peanut allergy, whereas Jewish children living in the U.K. avoid peanut and have ten times the rate of peanut allergy (Du Toit 2008).

Bamba is a snack, much like peanut-flavored Cheetos, which is being used to help expose infants to peanut earlier and more safely. Early exposure to other common food allergens has also been shown to decrease the rate of allergy.

This entire idea of introducing potentially allergic substances early is very counterintuitive and a little scary. When I was an Internal Medicine resident and then an Allergy and Immunology fellow, the mantra of the day was first, completely avoid feeding the allergic food to severely allergic children, and second, delay its introduction substantially. In fact, I delayed feeding these allergic foods to my own children because that is what a good mother would do.

Late one day, I returned home from work to find that *my mother had literally fed my daughter Katie every food allergen in one day*.

"Oh, my goodness! Is Katie all right? What will my colleagues say?"

But Katie was all right and my mother was more correct in her approach than either she or I knew at the time!

While it is definitely not the approach of the allergist-immunologist to introduce every highly allergic food all at once, we've learned that delaying solid foods, even the allergenic ones, is not necessarily the answer either. Of course, it is wise to get help for high-risk patients, including highly allergic children and children with asthma.

High-risk patients are also identified as those with wheezing at a young age, allergic parents or siblings, and those with multiple food allergies and eczema. Ongoing, regular, low-level exposure to allergic foods might decrease the risk of developing food allergy or additional food allergies. The parameters and the limits of this early exposure are still being investigated. A related but still important issue is this is an age when the type of exposure needs to be carefully monitored, as solid food can also be a choking hazard.

On the other hand, the reason many allergist-immunologists want to limit testing to the specific foods identified by patients as causing symptoms is that, if a patient does not eventually bring non-problematic foods back into their diet, strict avoidance and lack of exposure may erode food tolerance and potentially *increase* the risk of allergy over time.

Chapter 6

Recognize, Respond to, and Understand Anaphylaxis

Chapter Preview

- What are the signs and symptoms of anaphylaxis, the most severe allergic reaction?
- How to respond to an anaphylactic attack.
- Which medications to take for mild symptoms and which to take for severe symptoms.
- Essential tips on acquiring, storing, and using an epinephrine auto-injector.

Many other conditions can present with signs or symptoms of anaphylaxis, but following are the key signs of a serious allergic reaction that must be treated immediately (Kim 2011).

What Is Anaphylaxis?

Anaphylaxis is a severe respiratory problem caused by an allergic response of the immune system. Symptoms of anaphylaxis can appear literally within *seconds* of ingesting the food allergen or exposure to the allergen, but can be delayed a few hours after exposure. Reactions to food allergens usually appear within 30-60 minutes after consumption; reactions to parenteral (injected, infused, or implanted) medication or insect stings can occur even faster. Usually, symptoms of anaphylaxis that will go on to be more severe will present more quickly.

Most acute (short-term) allergic reactions are mild and self-limited, involving a single organ system, often the skin, with symptoms such as swelling of the lips or face, hives or welts, or tingling of the mouth.

Anaphylaxis is distinguished from a mild or moderate allergic reaction by the sudden involvement of two or more organ systems, manifesting with a variety of symptoms such as difficulty breathing, swelling of the tongue, swelling or tightness in the throat, wheezing, sudden persistent cough, abdominal pain, vomiting, and hypotension.

Anaphylaxis can also be diagnosed by the isolated involvement of the cardiovascular system in the setting of hypotension (severe drop in blood pressure) or cardiovascular collapse after exposure to a known allergen. Although isolated hypotension is a rare presentation of anaphylaxis, it often results in hospitalization and can be a marker of severity.

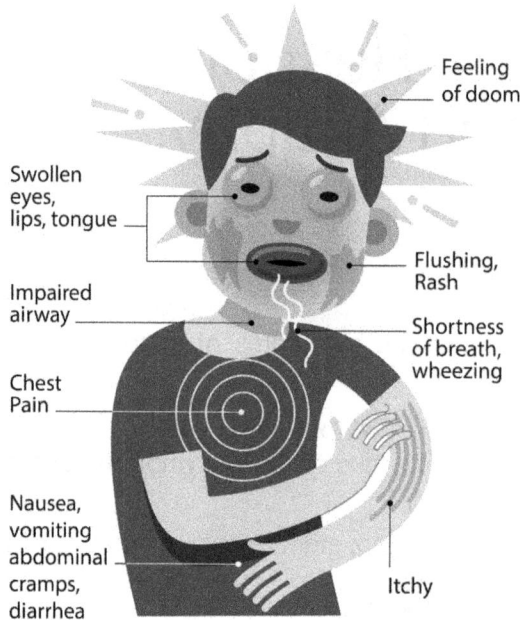

Feeling of doom

Swollen eyes, lips, tongue

Flushing, Rash

Impaired airway

Shortness of breath, wheezing

Chest Pain

Nausea, vomiting abdominal cramps, diarrhea

Itchy

Figure 13: Top symptoms of a severe allergic reaction.

Top Symptoms of an Allergic Reaction

There is no such thing as a *typical* allergic reaction. A person may experience one, two, several, or none of the common symptoms listed below. Further, the symptoms may occur generally in the following sequence, may overlap, or present in a completely different order. But it's still helpful to be aware of the key signs of an allergic reaction so you can help yourself or another person.

For example, the skin is often the first place symptoms of allergic reaction are visible, giving doctors and medics essential external signals about internal reactions. However, when a patient regularly uses antihistamines for upper respiratory symptoms, this drug may suppress the skin symptoms of a reaction, leaving medical personnel without those key visual signals and thus allowing a more severe allergic reaction to evolve.

1. Skin Rash

A red, hot, itchy skin rash is often the first visible symptom of an allergic reaction. 80-95% of patients with anaphylaxis also have skin symptoms (Mali 2012). Any allergen that can cause anaphylaxis can cause a skin rash.

2. Extreme Hay Fever

Red, watery eyes, nasal congestion, and other extreme hay fever symptoms may be an early sign of an allergic reaction. These may be the only symptoms. However, in a severe allergic reaction, these symptoms may be followed by flushing, shortness of breath, and loss of consciousness. Therefore, despite their mild nature, it is best not to underestimate these symptoms.

3. Red Eyes

Patients suffering from anaphylaxis may present with red, itchy, watery, bloodshot eyes. If you are experiencing this symptom in association with other anaphylaxis symptoms, you should seek medical attention as soon as possible.

4. Swelling (Edema)

Swelling is another common symptom of allergic reactions. Swelling signals that the immune system has been activated and an allergic reaction is about to occur or is occurring. The body parts—usually starting with the eyes, lips, hands, and face—become red, warm, and swollen due to fluids accumulating in those areas. While this may only be disfiguring, when this swelling occurs in the throat or tongue, impairing the airway, it can be life-threatening.

5. Breathing Difficulty

Respiratory system symptoms are among the most concerning symptoms of allergic reactions. *When swelling is visible externally, it may also be occurring internally.* A mild allergic reaction may cause nasal congestion, repeated sneezing, and a runny nose. A severe allergic reaction can cause the tongue and throat to swell, restricting the airway and making it difficult to swallow, wheezing of the lungs, increasing breathing difficulty, loss of consciousness, and death.

6. Gastrointestinal Upset

Allergic reactions can affect the entire digestive system, especially if the condition is a result of eating certain foods or taking certain medications. Symptoms can include severe cramps, nausea, diarrhea, and vomiting.

However, the same symptoms could be caused by a non-allergic reaction or other medical condition. For this reason, you need to visit a doctor to obtain a correct diagnosis of your child's reaction.

7. Cardiovascular Problems

Anaphylaxis can lead to cardiac and vascular symptoms. Allergic reactions flood the bloodstream with certain chemicals which cause the blood vessels to expand, leading to dizziness from a severe decrease in blood pressure.

8. Confusion

Confusion is the first neurologic symptom that appears during anaphylactic reactions. If your child starts feeling lightheaded, tell someone that he/she may be having an allergic reaction. An anaphylactic reaction can cause acute mental confusion, a loss of orientation, and an inability to describe things well.

9. Anxiety

Extreme anxiety, restlessness, and a desire to seek medical attention—even if the symptoms don't appear to warrant it—can signal the possibility of a severe anaphylactic reaction. The feelings associated with anaphylaxis are also described as a strong sense of impending doom.

When one of my patients said, "I need to call my mother; I think I am going to die," I took it seriously, although his visible symptoms weren't that severe at the time. Fortunately, I measured his blood pressure, which was too low to be read. Thankfully, quick intervention saved him. This is a good example of thoughts of impending doom. People who have had an anaphylactic reaction in the past can usually anticipate another episode when they feel this strong sensation.

10. Loss of Consciousness

Temporary loss of consciousness, whether partial or complete, can occur during an anaphylactic reaction, usually due to a sudden drop in blood pressure. The patient may feel lightheaded at first and then dizzy before they fall unconscious. So, if your child feels dizzy, tell someone close by that he/she may be about to have an anaphylactic reaction. While these symptoms are very severe, they can be a sign of vasovagal syndrome, which is a rapid drop in heart rate and blood pressure, typically brought on by an anxiety-provoking event (the sight of blood or the feeling of a needle injected into the arm, for example).

◆ ◆ ◆

How can I tell if someone is having an anaphylactic reaction?

Look for these signs, usually involving the nose, mouth, skin, or digestive system. Multiple symptoms may happen _very_ quickly and at the same time.

- Difficulty breathing.
- Rash or swollen lips.
- Signs of low blood pressure, such as a weak pulse, confusion, or loss of consciousness.
- Stomach symptoms, such as vomiting, diarrhea, and cramping.

How would you react to a SUDDEN REACTION after eating food?

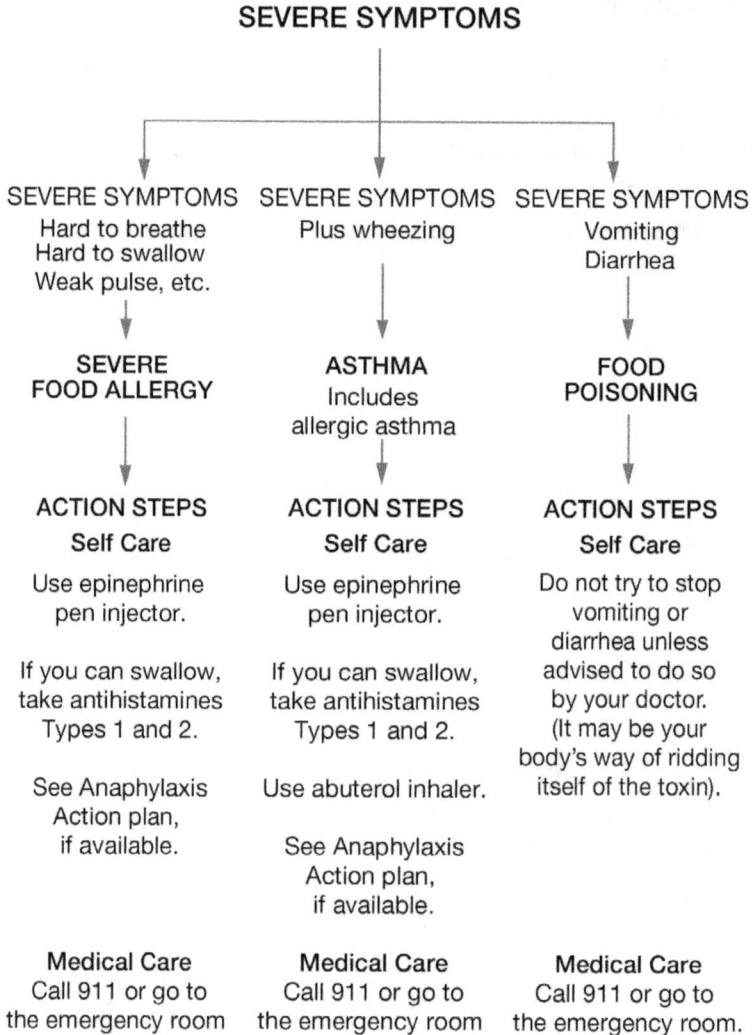

SEVERE SYMPTOMS

SEVERE SYMPTOMS	SEVERE SYMPTOMS	SEVERE SYMPTOMS
Hard to breathe Hard to swallow Weak pulse, etc.	Plus wheezing	Vomiting Diarrhea
SEVERE FOOD ALLERGY	**ASTHMA** Includes allergic asthma	**FOOD POISONING**
ACTION STEPS **Self Care**	**ACTION STEPS** **Self Care**	**ACTION STEPS** **Self Care**
Use epinephrine pen injector.	Use epinephrine pen injector.	Do not try to stop vomiting or diarrhea unless advised to do so by your doctor. (It may be your body's way of ridding itself of the toxin).
If you can swallow, take antihistamines Types 1 and 2.	If you can swallow, take antihistamines Types 1 and 2.	
See Anaphylaxis Action plan, if available.	Use abuterol inhaler. See Anaphylaxis Action plan, if available.	
Medical Care Call 911 or go to the emergency room	**Medical Care** Call 911 or go to the emergency room	**Medical Care** Call 911 or go to the emergency room.

Figure 14: Decision tree for various types of reactions.

What should I do if someone near me is going into anaphylactic shock?

If you are nearby when someone is having an anaphylactic reaction, call 911 or get medical help immediately. The person may need CPR as well.

MILD SYMPTOMS

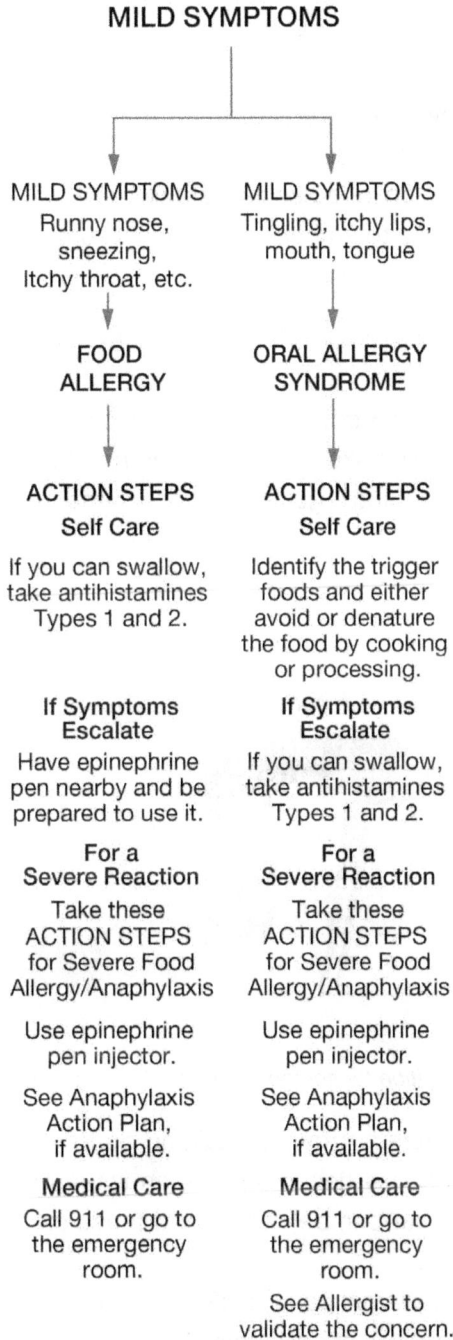

MILD SYMPTOMS	MILD SYMPTOMS
Runny nose, sneezing, Itchy throat, etc.	Tingling, itchy lips, mouth, tongue

FOOD ALLERGY	ORAL ALLERGY SYNDROME

ACTION STEPS

Self Care	Self Care
If you can swallow, take antihistamines Types 1 and 2.	Identify the trigger foods and either avoid or denature the food by cooking or processing.

If Symptoms Escalate	If Symptoms Escalate
Have epinephrine pen nearby and be prepared to use it.	If you can swallow, take antihistamines Types 1 and 2.

For a Severe Reaction	For a Severe Reaction
Take these ACTION STEPS for Severe Food Allergy/Anaphylaxis	Take these ACTION STEPS for Severe Food Allergy/Anaphylaxis
Use epinephrine pen injector.	Use epinephrine pen injector.
See Anaphylaxis Action Plan, if available.	See Anaphylaxis Action Plan, if available.

Medical Care	Medical Care
Call 911 or go to the emergency room.	Call 911 or go to the emergency room.
	See Allergist to validate the concern.

If this is your child and you know they are having an allergic reaction, it is time to enact your child's Anaphylaxis Action Plan: administer the epinephrine auto-injector while you are calling 911. If your child needs help, ask the 911 operator to coach you through the simple steps.

Patients with anaphylaxis should not sit, stand, or be placed in an upright position rapidly. Instead, as long as it is safe, they should be placed on their back with their lower extremities elevated as much as possible or, if they are experiencing respiratory distress or vomiting, they should be placed on their side with their lower extremities elevated, if possible and practical.

If you must move your child, do so *very slowly*. The extreme fluid shifts that occur during anaphylaxis can lead to empty ventricle syndrome, which can be fatal.

Other ways to help:

- If the person is unconscious, lay them on their side and open up their airway by lifting their chin.
- If the person is having trouble breathing, elevate the head and torso, but do so slowly, which will make it easier for them to breathe.
- If the person is breathing regularly, lay them either on their back or on their side.

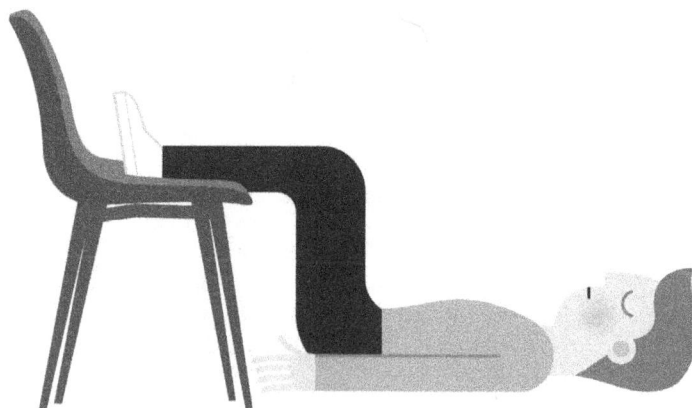

Figure 15: Recovery position for someone who had or is having an anaphylactic attack.

If your child has a severe allergy, maintaining good hydration habits is especially important for him/her because dehydration is an issue during anaphylaxis. The immense fluid shifts that occur can be deadly and these are exaggerated during initial treatment with epinephrine.

It's also important the allergic patient effectively manages any and all disease and medical conditions that would affect survival, such as asthma, other lung disease, and heart disease.

Prepare with an Anaphylaxis Action Plan

Every child with a severe food allergy and their parent(s) must know what to do in the event of a reaction. First, they need an Anaphylaxis Action Plan written by their allergist-immunologist (see my Anaphylaxis Action Plan in the Appendix). Second, they must know and understand the steps in the plan. Third, they must practice the steps so they are capable of responding correctly to a reaction.

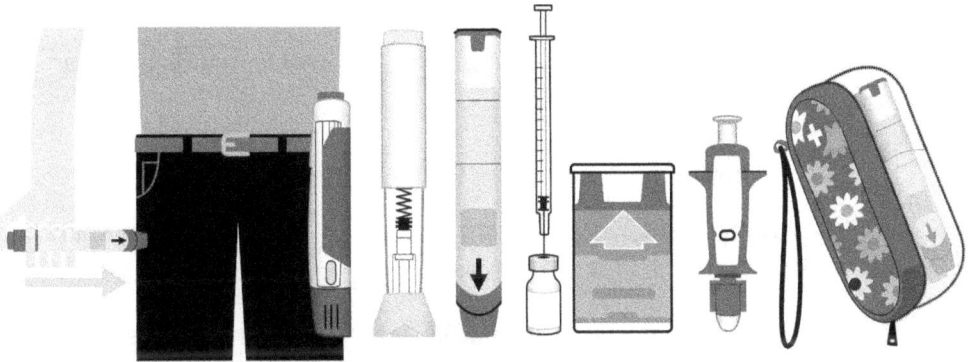

Figure 16: An epinephrine auto-injector can be injected into the thigh, or as your allergist recommends, directly through lightweight fabric. Do not try to inject through heavy fabric.

Know How to Use an Epinephrine Pen

It is very important that a child with food allergies has an epinephrine auto-injector readily available and knows how to use it, or a responsible and knowledgeable adult has immediate access and can administer the shot. Ideally, both should be the case. Carrying two epinephrine auto-injectors is even better, in case the allergic symptoms are severe.

The epinephrine injector should be practiced on a regular basis to determine if and when the child is capable of self-administration in an emergency and to build the child's comfort and confidence in using it. Every year when I am completing paperwork for my patient's schools and refilling epinephrine pens, I review how to use it and give my young patients a chance to show me how they would use their auto-injector.

Common brand names of epinephrine auto-injectors or epinephrine pens are Epipen, Auvi-Q, Symjepi, and Twinject.

Which Medications to Take for Mild Symptoms

If the food allergen has been consumed unintentionally and only mild symptoms result, I generally recommend the child/patient take one Type 1 antihistamine and one Type 2 antihistamine from the lists below. Take as directed by your child's allergist-immunologist until the symptoms are relieved. In my opinion, it is a good idea to put a dose appropriate for your child in the same protective carrying case you keep the epinephrine auto-injectors in so that there is no need to think about it in the middle of an emergency. There are several brands that are available as liquid pre-measured doses for children if they are not ready to swallow pills.

Type 1 antihistamines such as levocetirizine (Xyzal), cetirizine (Zyrtec), fexofenadine (Allegra), loratadine (Claritin) (note that loratadine has a delayed onset of action), or diphenhydramine (Benadryl).

Type 2 antihistamines such as famotidine (Pepcid), cimetidine (Tagamet), or nizatidine (Axid).

CAUTION: Be Ready for Escalating Symptoms

Also take the following precautionary steps so you and your child are prepared for a more severe allergic reaction should the mild allergic symptoms escalate:

1. Be sure to have the epinephrine auto-injector close at hand. In schools where the medication is secured in the nurse's office, move the patient to the nurse's office where the epinephrine auto-injector will be readily available.
2. If necessary, go to a medical facility where you can get help.

Avoid Regular Use of Antihistamines for Mild Allergic Symptoms

When mild symptoms of allergy such as a runny nose or mild itching appear after accidental exposure to the triggering substance, it is fine to take the prescribed antihistamine(s) and go to a medical facility where you can get help, if necessary.

Routine use of antihistamines for symptoms common to both allergies and non-allergies such as a runny nose (which can be caused by dust as well as an allergy) is not recommended. A better long-term solution to masking mild allergic symptoms with chronic use of antihistamines is to identify the food allergen and eliminate that food from your child's diet or pursue food oral immunotherapy.

Which Medications to Take for Severe Allergic Symptoms

If any of the more severe allergic symptoms develop such as shortness of breath, wheezing, chest tightness, swelling of the throat or tongue, extensive hives, flushing or faintness due to lowered blood pressure, call 911 immediately and administer the epinephrine auto-injector.

Know and understand your child's Anaphylaxis Action Plan before potential exposure of your child to his/her allergy. If you don't have one, ask your allergist-immunologist to design one as soon as possible (find my Anaphylaxis Action Plan in the Appendix.)

Use of Antihistamines for Severe Allergic Symptoms and Reactions

During an immediate allergic reaction (anaphylaxis), use of antihistamines is appropriate because antihistamine blocks histamine. However, unless anaphylactic symptoms continue to recur without warning or are not understood because the allergy has not been identified yet, there is no need to take antihistamines on a regular basis unless directed to do so by your child's allergist-immunologist.

All too often, new patients tell me they are "allergic to everything" and are regularly taking antihistamines, which seem benign but have definite potential side effects associated with them. Then, when I test, everything is negative (the patient does not have identifiable allergies). While antihistamines dry the nose and mouth out (which is a side effect, good only if it helps with allergy symptoms), there are other more direct and more appropriate ways of dealing with nonallergic symptoms, some of which may seem like allergy symptoms but, in these patients with no allergies, are not related to allergy.

Factors That Increase Risk of Death from a Severe Allergic Reaction

The difficult fact is that a severe allergic reaction can be fatal. However, addressing the following risk factors and other medical conditions that would negatively affect the outcome of a severe allergic reaction—such as dehydration—can lower the risk of death significantly. If any of the risk factors below are relevant to your child and are not under control, please return to your child's allergist-immunologist for a reassessment.

1. Delayed or omitted epinephrine treatment
2. Youth and inexperience – Teenagers and young adults are at highest risk for fatal anaphylaxis from risky behaviors based on their inability to understand cause and effect, lack of judgment, peer pressure, bullying, etc.
3. Pre-existing or poorly controlled asthma
4. Previously diagnosed food allergy
5. Lack of skin symptoms such as hives, flushing, and rashes
6. Use of alcohol
7. Denial of the allergic reaction symptoms
8. Dysfunctional family structure
9. Previous history of allergic reaction, especially if severe
10. Poor access to medical care
11. Overwhelmed parents (I personally fit into this category)

Food allergy is a primary cause of anaphylaxis. Therefore, immediate referral to a board-certified allergist-immunologist is not only important, it may also be lifesaving.

Important Notes about Your Child's Epinephrine Auto-Injector

- **Keep it nearby**

  Your child's epinephrine pen can only be helpful if you keep it with you and your child (or a responsible adult if you are not present), so _always_ keep one handy in a pocket, backpack, or purse. If your child has severe allergies and high risk of anaphylaxis, I strongly recommend you keep two pens with you and your child at all times. Your school may require this medication to be kept in the nurse's office along with your child's Anaphylaxis Action Plan. However, as soon as your child can reasonably give the epinephrine pen to himself/herself, I advocate keeping it in his/her backpack so it can be reached quickly.

- **Practice with the pen**

  Your child must be able to inject himself/herself with the epinephrine auto-injector without hesitation. While it is designed for very easy use, the circumstances in which it is needed are frightening, so practice is very important. Once your child's renewed prescription is refilled, practice using the old, expired pen on an orange or a grapefruit. Also, my office has a trainer pen you and your child can practice with during appointments.

- **Practice the process**

  Take your child's Anaphylaxis Action Plan and ask questions about various common scenarios: What would you do if you were in the lunchroom at school? What would you do if you were in class celebrating a birthday and you were given a cupcake? What if you were handed candy at Halloween? Ask your child these questions and see how he/she responds. If nothing else, it will give you an idea of your child's understanding of the situation and help you determine the level of responsibility you should assign to him/her. These are also great times for reviewing epinephrine pen use.

- **Smart storage**

  Store at room temperature. Do not expose an epinephrine auto-injector to extreme temperatures by storing it in your car during summer heat or winter cold. Do not store it in the refrigerator or in your car. Ideally, because it is most effective longest at room temperature, it is best kept in a purse or backpack for easy access.

- **Drugs that can reduce epinephrine's effectiveness**

  Medications that block the beta receptor, such as antihypertensive beta blockers or eye drop beta blockers for glaucoma, can render an epinephrine injection useless because it actually reduces resuscitation ability. Beta blockers should also be avoided because they reduce epinephrine's effectiveness and will make anaphylaxis more difficult to treat. Please make me or your child's allergist-immunologist aware if you or your child is taking one of these medications, so an alternate rescue medication can be prescribed.

- **Drugs that should be avoided**

  Certain medications typically used only by adults should be avoided when possible or used with extreme caution in people with unpredictable anaphylaxis, including angiotensin-converting enzyme inhibitors, beta blockers, angiotensin receptor blockers, monoamine oxidase inhibitors, and certain tricyclic antidepressants. These medications are known to exacerbate anaphylaxis symptoms or make resuscitation more challenging. In certain cases, such as surgery, patients may need to be exposed to an agent that places them at risk, in which case a pre-operative appointment with an allergist-immunologist is necessary.

- **Expiration date**

  Finally, remember that an epinephrine auto-injector, like any medication, has an expiration date. When this date is approaching, you should make an appointment to see me, renew your child's prescription, and update me on your progress.

  When you receive the epinephrine auto-injector from the pharmacy, make sure its expiration date is at least one year in the future *before* you leave the pharmacy counter. After you leave the counter, the medication will not be returnable.

  If you forget to have your child's prescription renewed, use your child's old pen if necessary. It may not be as effective as a new prescription, but it is better than nothing. I highly recommend you place the date on your calendar and also create a reminder one month ahead of time so you can make an appointment and get your child's new epinephrine on time.

  If your child is in school, consider getting the school district anaphylaxis paperwork ahead of time and meeting with your child's allergist-immunologist one month before the school year begins. I have seen epinephrine auto-injectors back-ordered during times when children are returning to school. Best not to be without one for the school year!

- **When and how to use your child's epinephrine auto-injector**

  When in doubt, use the epinephrine auto-injector and go immediately to the nearest emergency room for continued observation. If the first injection is working but your child's symptoms aren't significantly diminished, wait 15 seconds to 2 minutes after the first injection before using a second injector. If you use an epinephrine auto-injector—or even consider using one—go immediately to the nearest emergency room for continued observation.

  - The epinephrine auto-injector can be injected through light clothing such as jeans, slacks, or a skirt, but not through a heavy winter coat or multiple layers of clothing. Be careful about pockets (especially ones that are filled), seams, and folds in the clothing.
  - _Never_ remove your child to a bathroom to take off clothes and administer the epinephrine pen. First, it is not necessary. Second, it makes him/her invisible to others that may be able to help you or call for help.
  - Epinephrine takes only 15 seconds to 2 minutes to take effect. If symptoms continue to be severe and/or if new symptoms appear, use a second injector pen. At this point, if 911 has not been called, call 911.
  - Biphasic anaphylaxis, a recurrent anaphylaxis episode that can happen after a period of recovery, can be far worse than the first episode and is usually attributed to delayed or inadequate doses of epinephrine. Biphasic anaphylaxis is potentially life-threatening.
  - Great caution should be used in rising from a lying or seated position after using epinephrine, as this can worsen the already present and sometimes extreme fluid shifts of anaphylaxis. Epinephrine can temporarily increase blood pressure and heart rate (two reasons it is effective), but can increase the risk of a rhythm abnormality in patients who are prone to heart rhythm issues.
  - If you ever need to give your child epinephrine and/or visit an emergency room for a severe allergic response, make an appointment with your child's allergist-immunologist immediately afterward to review the situation.
  - Antihistamines are an appropriate response to a severe allergic reaction _after_ epinephrine and _if_ choking on a pill is not a possibility. Antihistamines do not work fast enough to counteract a severe and rapid allergic reaction and are definitely not an effective substitute for an epinephrine auto-injector. Epinephrine works very quickly in the very short time you have to avoid a potentially fatal allergic reaction.

VERY IMPORTANT: DON'T BE AFRAID TO USE A SECOND EPINEPHRINE PEN

If, after the first injection, your child still has an overwhelming sense of doom, cannot catch his/her breath, his/her airway is about to close, or passing out is imminent, use the second epinephrine injector immediately! Once your child cannot breathe because of a closed airway or passes out, especially if alone, the game is over.

The benefits of taking epinephrine for a potentially fatal allergic reaction _far outweigh_ the risks of epinephrine's possible side effects, such as transient high blood pressure, heart rhythm disturbance, fluid shifts, extreme dehydration, and electrolyte abnormalities.

Allergic Reactions are Specific to the IgE

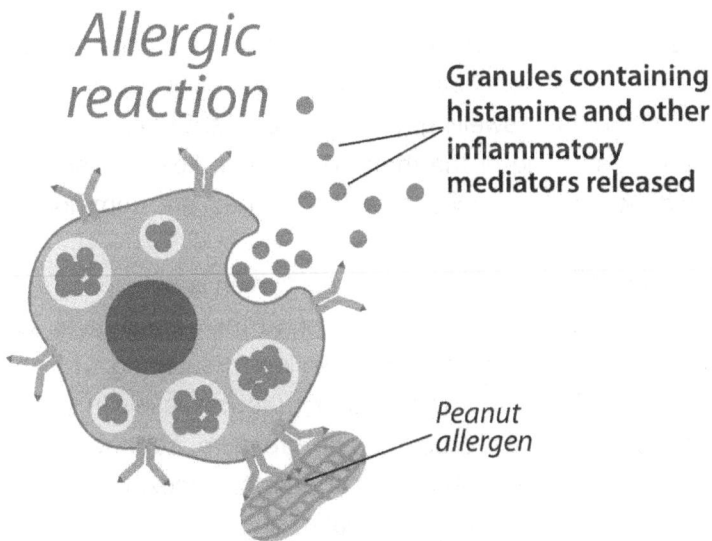

Figure 17: Allergic reaction to peanut with peanut protein latched onto peanut-specific flags.

There are two specific elements needed to cause an allergic reaction:

1. Presence of the triggering substance, antigen, or allergen: types of triggers range from environmental pollen to latex, medications, insects, and foods.
2. The body must be able to make allergic flags, the allergic antibody that recognizes the specific triggering substance. So, if your child is peanut allergic, your child is genetically capable of making a peanut-directed IgE (see fig. 17). The same is true if your child has a latex allergy; their body can make a latex-directed IgE. Note that the allergic flag for latex does not respond to bee venom.

Therefore, if your child is peanut allergic but successfully avoids peanut, he/she should not have an allergic reaction. The converse is also true: if your child is not peanut allergic, he/she can eat peanut and not have an allergic reaction.

However, there can be cross-reactivity in which the IgE for one allergen reacts to that of another allergen. For example, a patient with peanut allergy may also react to soybean because the IgE recognizes and sticks to the part of the protein that is very similar in each legume. In this cross-reactivity case, the protein is an albumin, the structure of which is about two-thirds the same in both legumes.

If the above two requirements—presence of allergy-specific allergic flag (IgE) and presence of the allergic substance—in this case, peanut and soybean—are met, the allergen is caught by peanut-specific IgEs on the mast cell (the master allergic cell), thus activating the cell.

The activated mast cell then releases chemical mediators that promote inflammation, such as histamines, leukotrienes, prostaglandins, and bradykinin, which cause familiar symptoms of nasal congestion such as post-nasal drip and runny nose; itchy, red, runny eyes; sinus pain, swelling, and pressure; shortness of breath, wheezing, and chest tightness; swelling of the throat or tongue; flushing, and hives. The term histamine should be familiar because antihistamines are commonly used to treat allergies.

Mast cells are located just beneath the skin (which is why allergist-immunologists perform skin tests—it is our chalkboard), around the vital organs, and around the blood vessels, which is why allergies can be so life-threatening. The chemical mediators of allergy cause leakage and dilation of the blood vessels in the body, which results in swelling, flushing, hives, drop in blood pressure, contraction of smooth muscles, nausea, vomiting, diarrhea, shortness of breath, wheezing, chest tightness, and/or swelling of the throat and tongue. If untreated or if it progresses too rapidly, allergic reaction can result in death.

To summarize, during a severe allergic reaction, your child's body mistakenly behaves as though the food or other allergen is a dangerous intruder and attacks it, sometimes at the body's own expense.

Eating Safely in Restaurants

Take precautions whenever you do not have control over your child's food. When eating out, bring your child's epinephrine pen and a friend who knows how to use it. Carry it with you—it can't help your child if it is in the car or at home—and *always* carry a phone.

Certain types of restaurants can be especially challenging to navigate for the food-allergic family. Buffets are notorious for cross-contamination and should probably be avoided. Caution is also recommended when considering restaurants where multiple dishes might be prepared without the pans or preparation utensils being changed.

It is safest to assume that restaurant workers and food preparers do not understand allergies or severe allergic reactions. Multiple studies have demonstrated that most restaurant workers did not understand the general principles of causes of food allergy like cross-contamination.

Cross-contamination occurs when an allergen (like milk or peanut) touches or is dropped into a nonallergic food. Many restaurant workers surveyed had the mistaken belief that if they removed the visible allergenic food by hand, the allergic person would be safe. Unfortunately, even though the allergic person cannot see the allergic food, the body can detect even microscopic amounts that are enough to potentially harm or cause death. Amazing, but very frightening!

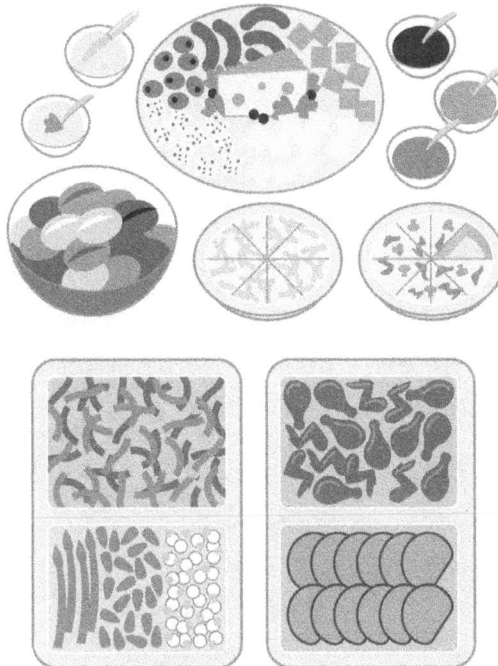

♦ ♦ ♦

This brings to mind a story; call it an early experiment that sealed my fate in becoming an allergist-immunologist. When I was little, I did not care for mushrooms. I noticed if I mentioned that I did not care for mushrooms to the wait staff at restaurants, they would still make it onto my plate. I decided to call myself allergic and when I asked to have them removed from the dish, I would always declare, "Please, because I am very allergic."

However, I would still see bits of mushroom on my plate. This speaks to the lack of understanding in restaurants about food allergies, which has improved but is definitely far from reliable.

The restaurant industry is slowly becoming more aware; some restaurants have designated kitchen areas, utensils, and pans specifically for allergic guests, but most do not. It only takes one new or poorly-trained waiter or kitchen staff member to unintentionally cause problems. (Unfortunately, I have seen this during my time as an allergist-immunologist.)

You must advocate for yourself and your child wherever you go. Ensure the allergic child knows to ask if their allergen is in the food. Even better, if the food is processed and from an unproven source, avoid it altogether. Also consider having your child wear a medical identification tag that warns of severe allergy. Examples are the MedicAlert and Allermates bracelet and necklace, which are labeled with allergies and emergency contact information in the event a child cannot speak or advocate for himself or herself.

♦ ♦ ♦

Chapter 7

Insights Into Children's Food Allergies

Chapter Preview

- What are the most common food allergies children experience?
- What is the likelihood of my child outgrowing their allergy?
- What are the cross-reactive foods about which we should know?

Top Nine Most Common Food Allergens

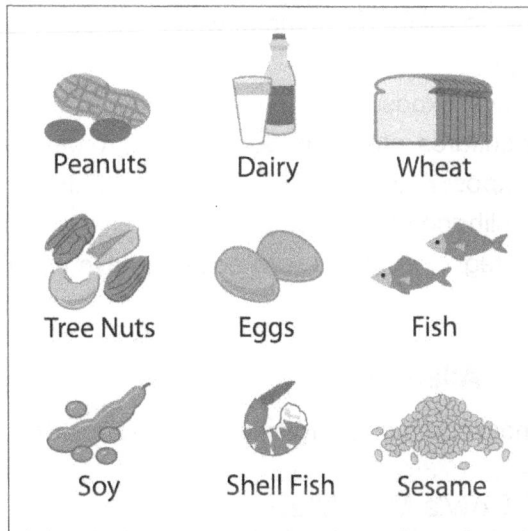

Peanuts   Dairy   Wheat

Tree Nuts   Eggs   Fish

Soy   Shell Fish   Sesame

Figure 18: Top nine most common food allergens.

Which Common Food Allergies Are Most Likely to Be Outgrown?

While cow's milk and egg are among the most common allergies of childhood, they are also the most likely to be outgrown. On the other hand, allergies to foods such as peanut, tree nuts, fish, and shellfish are much less likely to be outgrown.

The severity and ability to outgrow the allergy may be at least partially dependent on the lability (the ability or likelihood of a substance or compound to change or break down easily, rapidly, or continually) and stability of the antigen. For example, if a child has an allergy to the proteins in dairy curds (the more stable cow's milk proteins), this often portends an increased rate of severe reaction to all forms of milk and a decreased likelihood of outgrowing the allergy with age.

Similarly, if the proteins in egg whites and egg yolks are heat stable and the allergy is associated with an inability to tolerate baked egg products, there is a decreased likelihood of outgrowing the allergy with age (Unsworth 2014).

In contrast, if the stability of the protein in the whey of cow's milk is low, and extensively heated milk, such as that present in baked products, can be tolerated, there is a greater likelihood of outgrowing the allergy.

Other factors that affect the ability to outgrow a food allergy:

- Age - Younger patients that present earlier and with more allergies tend to acquire more food and environmental allergies as they age.
- Exposure - Technically, your child needs to be exposed to the allergen a second time to have an allergy, for reasons already described.
- Gut maturity - Immaturity of the gut and the immune system makes the infant more vulnerable to allergens, some of which will be outgrown as the immune system develops.
- Repeated low level exposure—such as in food oral immunotherapy as well as the way some cultures introduce foods—tends to decrease allergy.
- Route of first exposure tends to be important. Inhaling, for example, tends to increase the likelihood of allergy.
- Skin and gut integrity. Patients with eczema have a high rate of increase of allergies.

Common Childhood Allergies

Listed below are the most common allergies and some considerations unique to each.

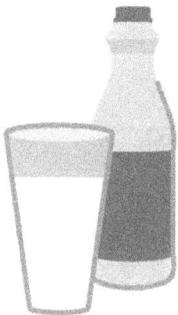

Cow's Milk Allergy

Cross-reactivity

Some patients with cow's milk allergy are sensitized to other foods that have similar proteins, as follows:

9-10% of patients also react to beef

90% of patients also react to other mammalian milks such as that of goat and sheep

18-60% of patients react to mammalian milks such as that of horse, donkey, camel, and human

50% of patients also have soy allergy

Cow's milk allergy affects 0.25-4.9% of the population (Warren 2019).

Potential for development of tolerance

Cow's milk allergy resolves over time/with age for a significant number of patients, as follows:

19% of patients by age 4

64% of patients by age 12

79% of patients by age 16

When to reassess

Recommended yearly due to the high and rapid rate of developing tolerance.

Frequent consumption speeds tolerance

Diets that include the regular consumption of extensively heated (baked) cow's milk (≥ 5 times per month) increase the development of tolerance four times faster than in children who eat baked cow's milk less frequently (<5 times per month). The ability to tolerate baked cow's milk in a muffin is also predictive of a faster rate of tolerance development to less-cooked cow's milk, as in warmed milk for cocoa.

Baby formula made of extensively hydrolyzed casein is an alternative to cow's milk for infants and very young children and can be used to attempt tolerance induction.

What is an extensively hydrolysed formula?

In most cases where breastfeeding is not an option for infants with cow's milk protein allergy (CMPA), guidelines recommend an extensively hydrolysed formula (eHF) as appropriate first-line dietary management, with the ultimate goal being to ensure normal growth and symptom relief. These guidelines also state that an eHF should be well-tolerated by at least 90% of infants with CMPA (with a 95% confidence interval).

Heating milk reduces allergic reaction for some patients

About 75% of milk-allergic patients can tolerate extensively heated cow's milk, as in a muffin, but not tolerate lightly heated cow's milk, such as when warmed for hot cocoa.

More precisely, low-heat pasteurization (75C/167F for 15 seconds) of store-bought milks is not enough to reduce allergenicity. However, high heat treatment (121C/250F for 20 minutes) destroys the allergenicity of whey and decreases that of casein or curd.

Cow's milk protein-induced iron deficiency

Cow's milk protein-induced iron deficiency is a late reaction to cow's milk. As the name implies, it results in iron deficiency in infancy. It presents at less than 12 months old. Eliminating cow's milk results in resolution. This condition has become exceptionally rare.

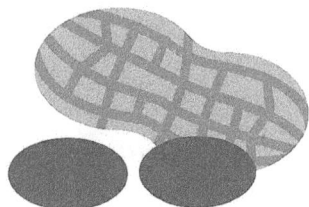

Peanut Allergy

Cross-reactivity

With peanut allergy, there is a 5% likelihood of allergy to other legumes such as peas, lentils, and beans. It affects 1.5-3 % of the population (Warren 2019).

Potential for development of tolerance

Peanut allergy resolves in 22% of patients by age four.

When to reassess

Recommended every two years due to the lower rate of remission.

See the Appendix for muffin recipes for children with milk and egg allergies who can tolerate baked milk and baked egg. These can be used to attempt to build tolerance to raw milk and raw egg slowly over time.

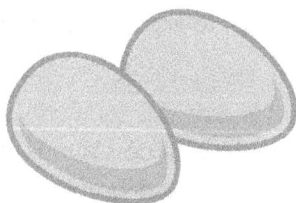

Egg Allergy

Cross-reactivity

With a chicken egg allergy, it's very common for the patient to react to other bird eggs. 22-32% of patients also react to chicken meat. Egg allergy affects 2% of the population (Warren 2019).

Potential for development of tolerance

When the egg-specific IgE is <2 kUa/L, tolerance to egg occurs in:

11% of patients by age 4

26% of patients by age 6

53% of patients by age 10

82% of patients by age 16

The COFAR group has a calculator that helps predict the probability of outgrowing egg allergy (http://cofargroup.org, Egg Allergy Resolution Calculator).

Heating egg reduces allergic reaction for some patients

38-50% of patients can tolerate extensively heated egg, such as in a muffin, but not lightly heated egg, such as in French toast or a scrambled egg, which should be avoided.

Diets with regular consumption of extensively heated (baked) egg (≥5 times per month) seem to increase the development of tolerance four times faster than those who eat baked egg less frequently (<5 times per month). The ability to tolerate baked egg (a muffin) is also predictive of a faster rate of tolerance than less-cooked egg (on French toast).

When to reassess

Recommended yearly due to greater likelihood of developing tolerance.

Vaccination in egg-allergic patients per the Centers for Disease Control

People with a history of egg allergy who have experienced only hives or less severe symptoms after exposure to egg should receive the flu vaccine. Any licensed and recommended flu vaccine that is otherwise appropriate for the recipient's age and health status may be used.

Those individuals who report having had reactions to egg involving symptoms other than hives—such as angioedema, respiratory distress, lightheadedness, re-current emesis, or who required epinephrine or another emergency medical inter-vention—may similarly receive any licensed and recommended flu vaccine that is otherwise appropriate for the recipient's age and health status, but they should be observed by an allergist or other health care professional able to recognize and man-age severe allergies (CDC).

A history of severe or life-threatening allergic reaction to a flu vaccine is a contra-indication to future receipt of the vaccine (CDC 2022).

The COFAR group has calculators that help predict the probability of outgrowing both cow's milk allergy and egg allergy (http://cofargroup.org).

The Allergen Labeling and Consumer Protection Act (FALCPA) of 2004 regulates labeling of products that "contain" the major allergens, including cow's milk, but does not regulate terms "may contain" or "manufactured on equipment with" (http://www.fda.gov/food/foodsafety/foodallergies). Essentially, intentional ingredient addition, as in a recipe, is covered by this act but unintentional addition (e.g., a worker moving from a processing/production line that contains the allergic substance to one that does not, thereby accidentally cross-contaminating the allergy-free production line) is not within the scope of this labeling.

What this means to you and your child is that any product labeled "may contain" or "manufactured on equipment with" may be processed with excellent quality control and all efforts made to keep foods free of allergic ingredients. However, it's simply impossible to control every possibility of cross-contamination and there is an inherent risk in consuming that processed food. While, most of the time, you may find that this is not an issue, it may occur during the processing and packaging of specific lots.

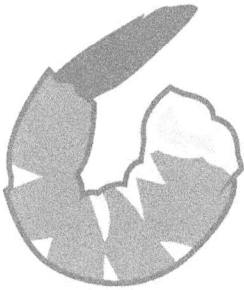

Shellfish Allergy

Shellfish are one of the most common food allergens and are divided into two groups, crustaceans and mollusks. A child's allergy to crustacean shellfish (shrimp, lobster, crayfish, crab) doesn't necessarily mean they are allergic to mollusk shellfish (mussels, oysters, scallops, squid, snail). However, there is a high percentage of cross-reactivity between the groups, as you'll read below. There is also a high likelihood of cross-contamination between types of shellfish, mollusks, and finned fish at the market and during preparation.

Cross-reactivity

With crustacean shellfish allergy, the level of protein cross-reactivity with mollusks is 75%, but the actual level of clinical mollusk allergy is 14%. There is also cross reactivity with the tropomyosin of other arthropods, such as cockroaches and dust mites. Shellfish allergy affects 2.3% of the population (Warren 2019).

Potential for development of tolerance

Less than 20% of patients resolve their shellfish allergy.

When to reassess

Recommended every two years due to the lower rate of tolerance development, or consider it a permanent diagnosis.

Note: Regarding shellfish-allergic patients, there is not an increased risk of reaction to radiocontrast media and no documented relationship between anaphylactic reactions to radiocontrast media and allergy to fish, crustacean shellfish, or iodine.

Soy Allergy

Cross-reactivity

With soy allergy, reactivity to cow's milk coexists in 50% of patients. Five percent of peanut-allergic patients are also allergic to other legumes, such as peas, lentils, and

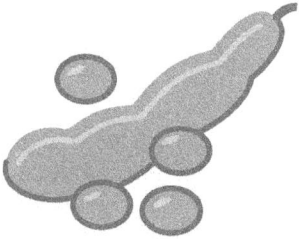

beans, including soybeans. Soy allergy affects about 3% of the population (Warren 2019).

Potential for development of tolerance

Soy allergy may resolve in:
29% by 4 years
45-67% by 6 years
69% by 10 years

When to reassess

Reassessment is recommended every year.

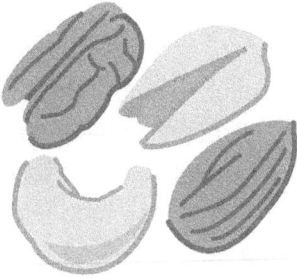

Tree Nut Allergy

Cross-reactivity

With tree nut allergy, there is a 37% likelihood of allergy to other tree nuts. It affects 1-2% of the population (Warren 2019).

Potential for development of tolerance

Tree nut allergy resolves in 10% of patients.

When to reassess

Recommended every two years due to the lower rate of tolerance development.

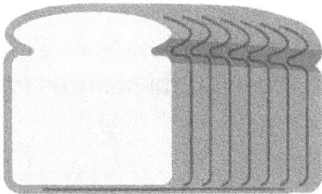

Wheat Allergy

Cross-reactivity

With wheat allergy, there is a 20-21% likelihood of allergy to other grains such as rye or barley. Wheat allergy affects 0.5-9% of the population (Warren 2019).

Potential for development of tolerance

There is a 50% chance of resolution of wheat allergies by seven years old.

When to reassess

Recommended every 12-18 months due to the rate of tolerance development.

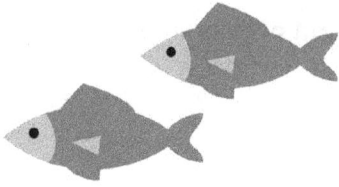

Fish Allergy

Cross-reactivity

With fish allergy, there is a 50% likelihood of being allergic to other fish and to frogs. Fish allergy affects 0.1-0.5% of the population (Warren 2019).

There are cases of allergy after consuming the fish parasite *Anisakis simplex* on contaminated fish. As well, fish that are decayed or even slightly aged, producing histamine, can create scombroid poisoning, which is an adverse response, not an allergy.

Potential for development of tolerance

Fish allergy resolves in a little less than 20% of patients.

Watch for surprise products that may contain fish, including gelatin, barbeque sauce, caponata, Worcestershire sauce, imitation fish and shellfish, and Caesar dressing. Also be aware that certain cuisines are renowned for use of fish-based seasonings: African, Thai, Filipino, Vietnamese, Cambodian, Laotian, Myanmar, Indonesian, and Chinese. Finned fish allergy and shellfish allergy are unrelated.

When to reassess

Recommended every two years due to the lower rate of tolerance development.

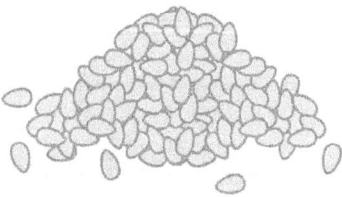

Sesame Allergy

Cross-reactivity

With sesame seed allergy, there is likelihood of cross-reactivity to poppy seeds, mustard seeds, and other seeds. The statistical likelihood of cross-reactivity has not been fully assessed at this time.

As of January 1, 2023, sesame seed allergy will be acknowledged as one of the most common allergens and labeling will be required as per FALCPA. Sesame allergy affects 0.23% of the population (Warren 2019).

Potential for development of tolerance

Only 27.1% of sesame-allergic children will eventually become tolerant (Gupta 2013).

When to reassess

Recommended every two years due to the lower rate of development of tolerance.

Other Food Allergens

Other priority food allergens associated with severe allergic reactions include buckwheat, lupin, celery, molluscum shellfish, and mustard.

Other Important Food Reactions

Other important non IgE-mediated reactions to food include cutaneous reactions such as eczema (atopic dermatitis), allergic contact dermatitis (a form of eczema), and contact hives.

Researchers have suggested that colic, gastroesophageal reflux, and constipation might be caused by food allergy in a small subset of patients (Sunkara 2019).

Chapter 8

The Many Swollen Faces of Angioedema

Chapter Preview

- What is angioedema and what are its most concerning symptoms?
- What are the causes of angioedema?
- Which medications are most helpful for allergic angioedema?

Angioedema is a skin condition that can result from an allergy, an inherited condition, or an autoimmune condition. Allergic triggers of angioedema include drugs; foods or food additives; inhalation, ingestion of, or contact with allergic substances such as tree, grass, and weed pollen; dog, cat, and animal dander; mold spores; medications; and insects.

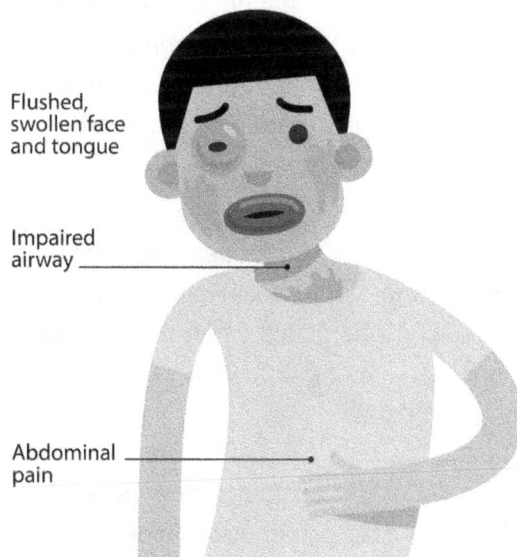

Flushed, swollen face and tongue

Impaired airway

Abdominal pain

Figure 19: Angioedema symptoms.

Angioedema is the swelling of the deeper layers of the skin, caused by a buildup of fluid. The symptoms of angioedema can affect any part of the body, but swelling usually affects the eyes, lips, genitals, hands, and feet. Many people with angioedema also experience urticaria (hives), a raised, red, itchy rash that appears on the skin.

Angioedema may include other symptoms such as difficulty breathing, red and irritated eyes, abdominal pain, a general unwell feeling, diarrhea, dizziness, and fainting. If your child has experienced angioedema, please contact your child's allergist-immunologist for testing and treatment. We might perform allergy testing, especially if you suspect that your child has an allergy or we suspect an allergy after we hear your child's medical history.

If there is one episode, the triggering factor is obvious, or the angioedema lasts less than six weeks, your child's symptoms were probably the result of an allergy. If there is no clear cause or the condition continues for more than six weeks, the cause is usually autoimmune. Sometimes, it is difficult even for an expert to determine this distinction.

However, what I've found is this: If the pattern is obvious, the cause is obvious. For example, some patients tell me, "I started using X and the swelling or hives started. Therefore, the swelling or hives must be from X."

Well, that usually *is* it! When the condition is chronic, it is usually related to an autoimmune condition. If the symptoms are less clear, they come and go without a clear pattern, or are less clearly linked, this tends to be the case.

Some people develop angioedema in response to cold temperatures, contact with a cold object (like an ice cube), sweating, sun exposure, scratching, heat, pressure, vibration, and water. This subtype of autoimmune angioedema is very similar to chronic idiopathic urticaria (hives), but in areas where the subcutaneous tissue is thinner so the swelling is not recognized as discrete hives.

Allergic Angioedema

Allergy is the most common cause of angioedema and the easiest problem to solve, so we check for allergies first. In a typical allergic reaction, mast cells release histamine and other allergy-causing chemicals when they recognize IgE attached to an allergic substance like shellfish (see fig. 20). This triggers mast cells to release histamine and allergy-causing chemicals.

Just about anything that causes an allergic reaction can result in angioedema. This includes food. The most common foods that cause anaphylaxis and food allergies in general are the same that can cause angioedema. As a matter of fact, angioedema can be one of the symptoms seen in cases of anaphylaxis.

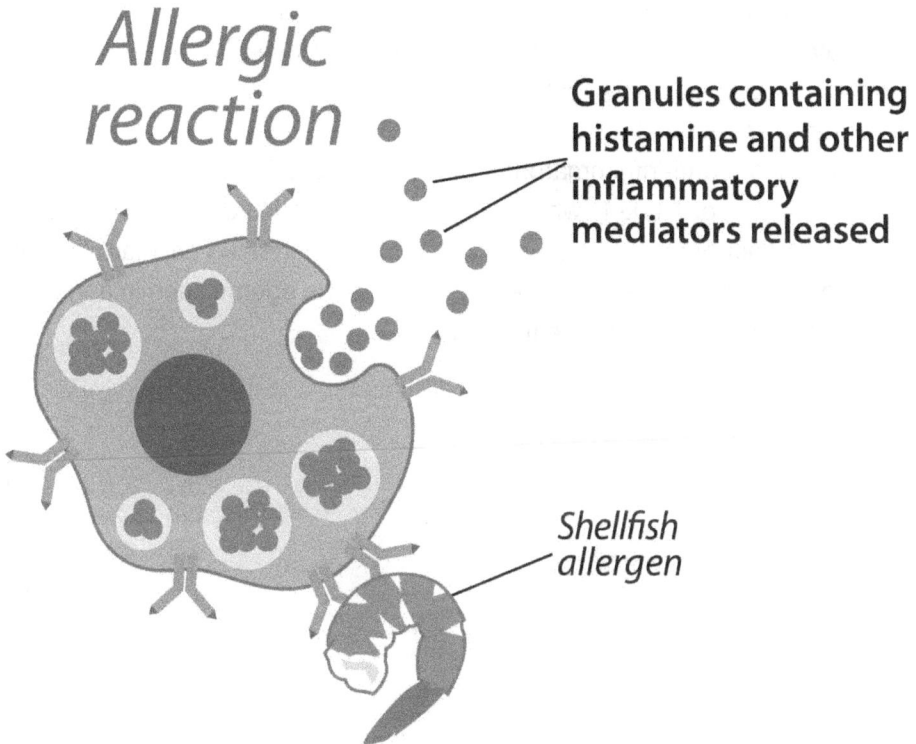

Figure 20: The mast cell recognizes allergies, seen here as shellfish, resulting in the stimulation of cell mechanisms that culminate in the release of histamine as well as other mediators of the allergic response.

Medication-Induced Angioedema

NSAIDs

Some patients with angioedema experience an exacerbation of symptoms on ingestion of aspirin or non-steroidal anti-inflammatory drugs (like naproxen, ibuprofen, aspirin, or indomethacin) or opioid analgesics (like hydrocodone or oxycodone). Therefore, it is important for these patients to avoid these drugs when possible.

Other mechanisms also cause symptoms that look like allergies. For example, opioids have their own receptor on the master allergic cell (called the opioid receptor). Any opioid can stimulate that receptor, causing it to release histamine and other mediators that are generally attributed to allergy.

Non-steroidal anti-inflammatories (NSAIDs) block an enzyme known as Cyclooxygenase-1 or COX-1, which diverts pathways inside allergenic cells to one that causes bronchoconstriction, vasoconstriction, increased capillary leakage, fluid leakage from blood vessels, and swelling, such as the edema seen in angioedema (in the absence of a true allergy) (see fig. 21).

Inflammation and NSAIDs

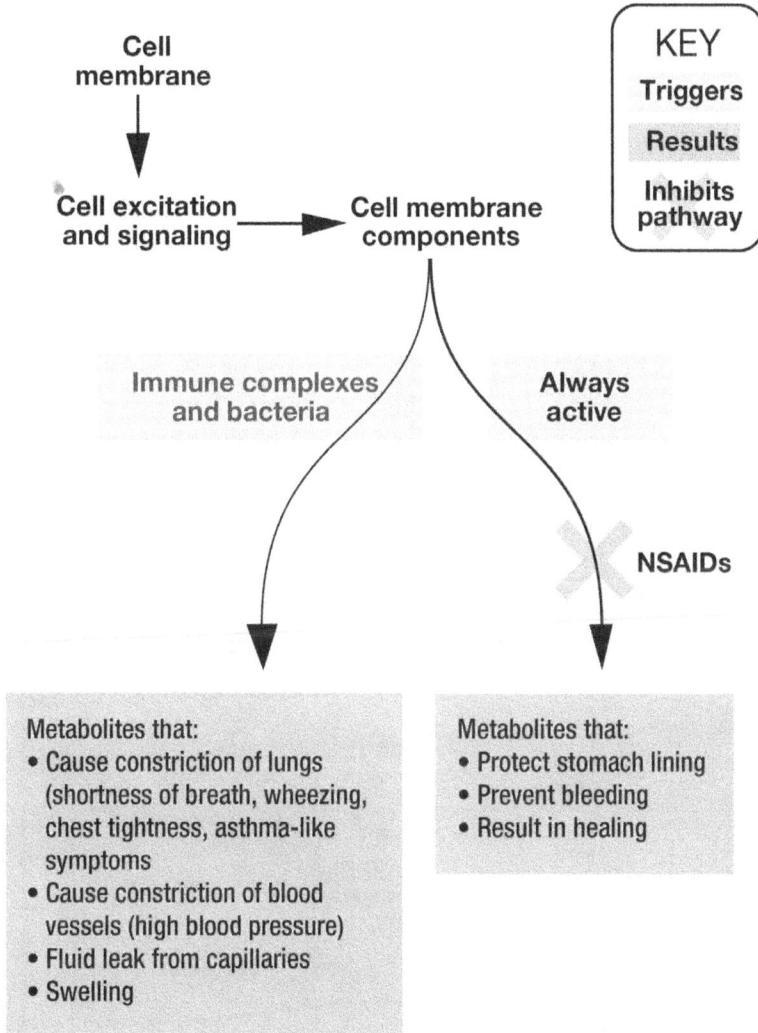

Figure 21: Non-steroidal anti-inflammatories (NSAIDs) block an enzyme known as Cyclooxygenase-1 or COX-1, which diverts pathways inside allergenic cells to ones that result in bronchoconstriction, vasoconstriction, increased capillary leakage, fluid leakage from blood vessels, and swelling, such as the edema seen in angioedema.

Normal Coagulation and Complement Pathways

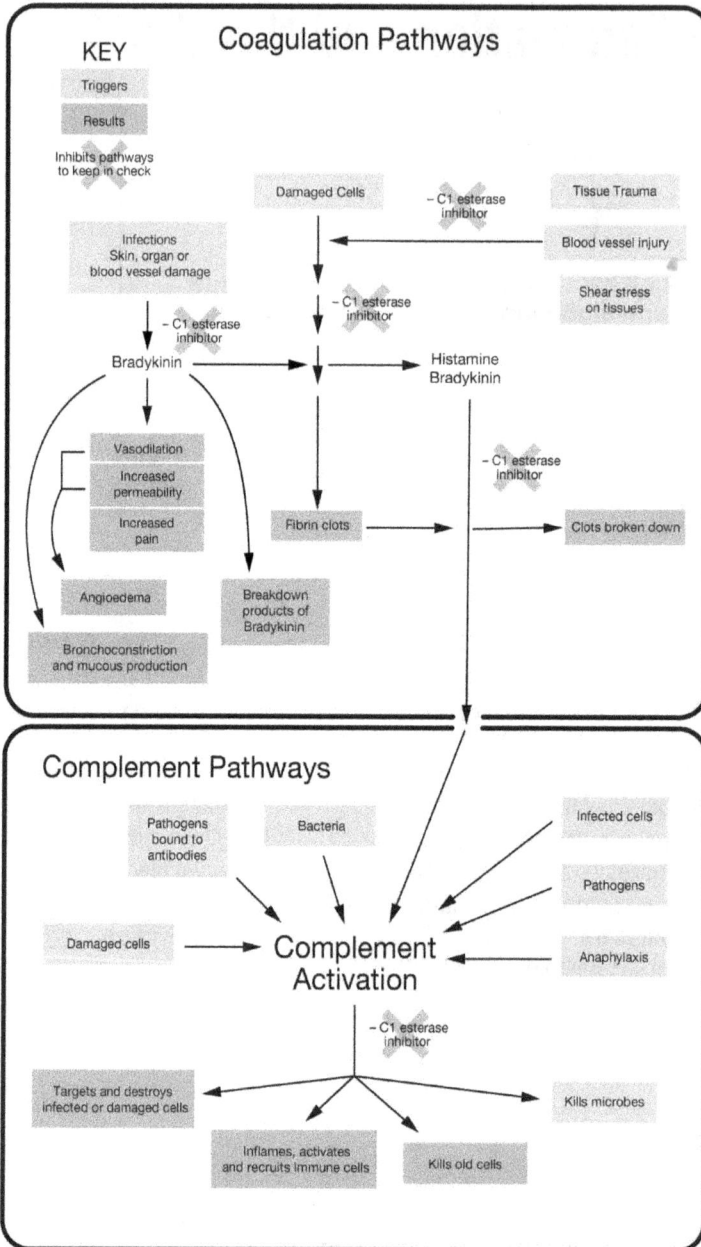

Figure 22: The normal coagulation and complement pathways. Noted are the parts of the pathway that C1 esterase inhibits, keeping them in check. While bradykinin and histamine seem to have many negative effects, during inflammation, these effects help the immune system fight infection. For example, when not kept under control, vasodilation and increased permeability would seem bad. However, this also helps immune cells get to where they need to be.

Ace Inhibitor Effect

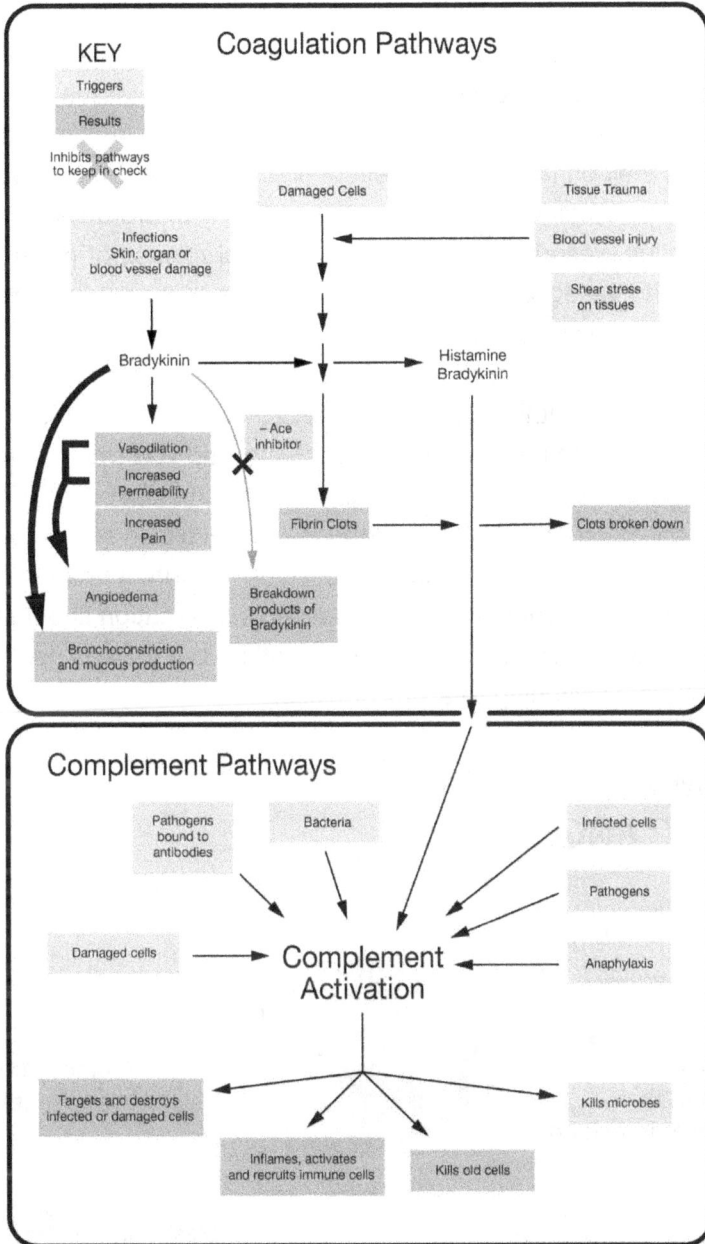

Figure 23: The Coagulation and Complement pathways under the effects of an ACE inhibitor. Instead of being broken down into harmless and inactive products, bradykinin is produced unchecked, causing vasodilation, increased permeability, and angioedema.

ACE Inhibitors and ARBs

Patients responding to medications with swelling or angioedema, especially of the throat and tongue, should also avoid medications of the angiotensin-converting enzyme (ACE) inhibitor or angiotensin receptor blocker (ARB) classes, typically used for blood pressure control and sometimes for kidney protection in diabetes.

In addition to their primary blocking effect on the angiotensin pathway, ACE inhibitors and ARBs also block degradation of substance P and bradykinin, which cause bronchoconstriction, vasodilation, pain, itching, local release of histamine, and ultimately leakage and vasodilation of the blood vessels that contribute to the swelling and pain of angioedema (see fig. 23).

It is important to understand that this reaction can occur at any time while on these medications, be it within two days or after 20 years. This seems counterintuitive if you're thinking about immediate allergic reactions, and you would be correct. While these medications can also cause an allergic reaction, in most cases the angioedema is caused by a diversion of a chemical pathway that results in swelling.

While these are excellent medications for hypertension, if unanticipated side effects such as angioedema and swelling appear, this medication should be discontinued. Some patients can tolerate a similar medication, but there is risk of recurrence, as well as a risk from switching to a similar class.

AUTOIMMUNE FORM of CHRONIC ANGIOEDEMA

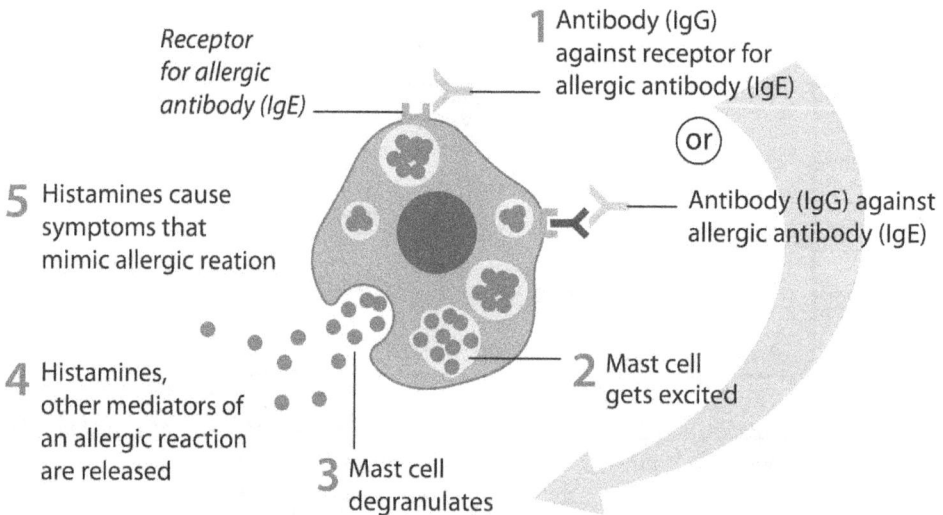

Figure 24: Mast cell triggered by auto-immune antibodies, causing angioedema. The most common causes of autoimmune angioedema result from auto-antibodies bound to the receptor for the antibody IgE (the allergic antibody) on mast cells or auto-antibodies.

Hereditary and Acquired Angioedema

The inherited and acquired forms of angioedema are not the result of allergy and therefore are not easily tested. Typically, some form of autoimmune disease, such as thyroid disease, rheumatoid arthritis, or vitiligo, has been noted in the patient or a family member. Acquired angioedema can also be caused by cancer.

Basic Understanding of Autoimmune Diseases

Auto-antibodies are antibodies directed against self. If they are not eliminated by the "checks and balances" of the immune system, auto-antibodies can lead to self-destruction. This is how many autoimmune diseases cause so many health challenges. That is, many of them have auto-antibodies in common. The reality is that most of us make auto-antibodies. But most of the time, they are destroyed by the immune system or do not result in substantive damage. When they do, however, they can result in diseases like thyroiditis, lupus, rheumatoid arthritis, and, of the conditions covered in this book, angioedema and hives. In these cases, it is the allergic cells that are the target of the auto-antibodies. When those auto-antibodies activate the allergic cells, causing them to release histamine and the other allergic mediators, the result is hives or angioedema (see fig. 24).

Hereditary Angioedema

Lack of or decreased activity of C1 esterase inhibitor causes hereditary angioedema (HAE), Type I or Type II, respectively. C1 esterase inhibitors work on important inflammatory reactions to reduce the amount of bradykinin and other mediators that cause inflammation and swelling (see figs. 25 and 26). When C1 esterase inhibitors are missing or dysfunctional, there is no brake in place for bradykinin production. Therefore, if these pathways are activated by events such as trauma, stress, surgery, infection, and so forth, patients with HAE tend to swell.

Type III angioedema is thought to be caused by mutations in a blood protein known as Factor XII. This type of angioedema occurs in women and is estrogen-responsive, so states such as pregnancy and oral contraception use precipitate attacks. There is no abnormality of C1 esterase in Type III HAE.

Normal Coagulation and Complement Pathways

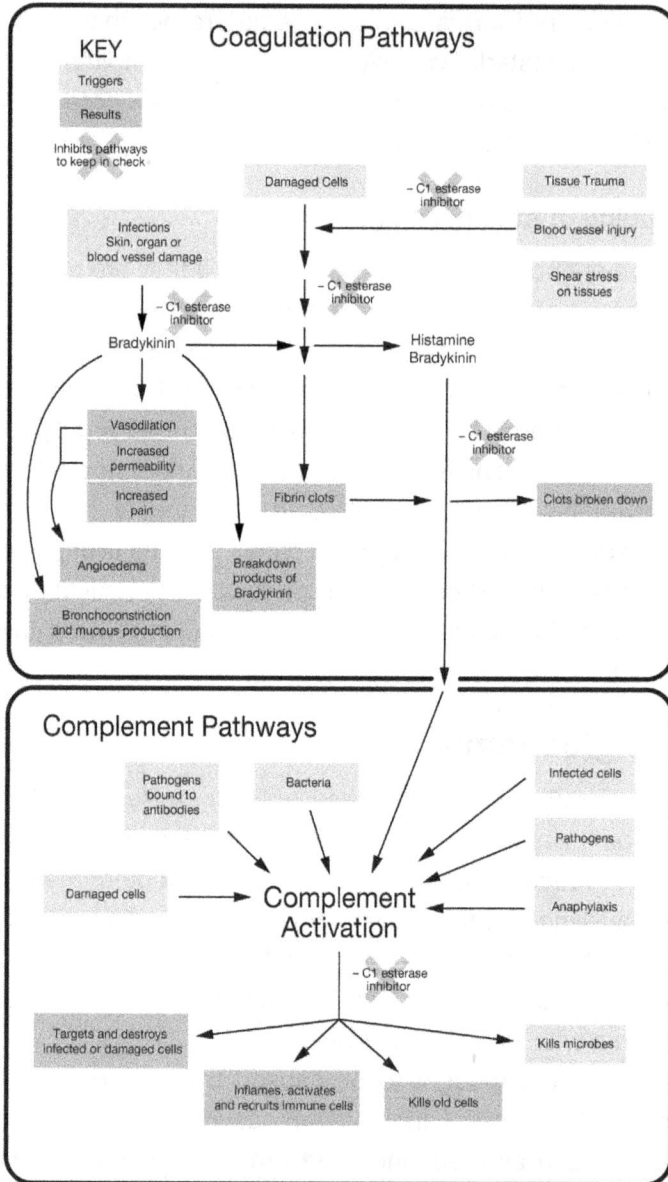

Figure 25: The normal coagulation and complement pathways. Noted are the parts of the pathway that C1 esterase inhibits, keeping them in check. While bradykinin and histamine seem to have many negative effects, during inflammation, these effects help the immune system fight infection. For example, when not kept under control, vasodilation and increased permeability would seem bad. However, this also helps immune cells get to where they need to be.

Absence of C₁ esterase inhibitor (function or protein)

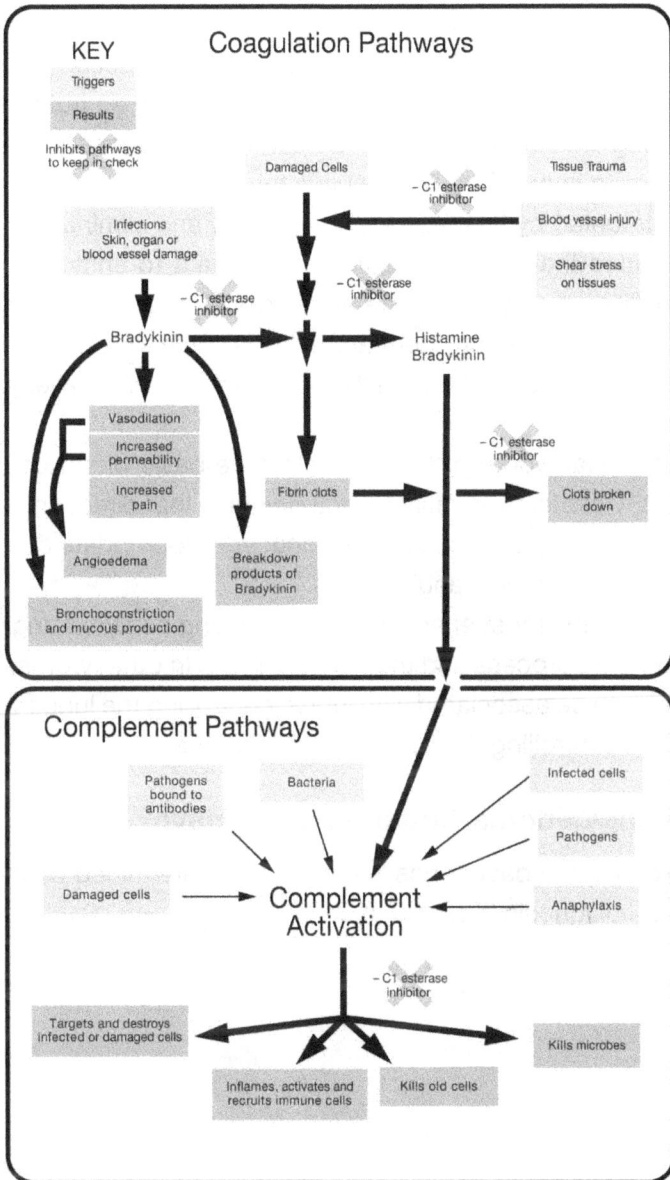

Figure 26: Hereditary angioedema, caused by absence of C1 esterase inhibitor function or protein. Compare this figure with Figure 12, the normal coagulation and complement pathways, with C1 esterase inhibitor function intact, keeping many of these processes in check. Then review the differences in this figure, where the C1 esterase inhibitor function is gone, allowing many of these processes to continue unchecked, resulting in increased vasodilation, increased permeability and therefore angioedema.

Acquired Angioedema

Acquired angioedema is caused by an acquired deficiency of the C1 esterase inhibitor. This results in the same inappropriate activation of the reaction that causes an unopposed increase in bradykinin. This is typically caused by an autoimmune process in which neutralizing antibodies target the C1 esterase inhibitor protein that is associated with several autoimmunities. The result is the same as C1 esterase protein deficiency, as this is targeted by the neutralizing antibody and eliminated (see Figure 26).

Any circumstance that causes the immune system to shift into high gear and make excess antibodies may cause the angioedema to flare. Trigger processes include some forms of lymphoma, dermatomyositis, other rheumatologist diseases, cancer, etc. The acquired form of angioedema is not the result of allergy and therefore is not easily tested.

As part of the initial work-up, tests may include basic blood counts as well as kidney, liver, and thyroid tests. If initial testing points in that direction, we may test for signs of other autoimmune diseases or ask about age-appropriate cancer screenings that tend to accompany chronic angioedema.

In my experience, the most effective form of treating acquired angioedema is determining the triggering process and then controlling it. In other words, if the acquired angioedema seems to be associated with lupus, controlling the lupus with medication would also result in controlling the acquired angioedema.

What Type of Angioedema Could My Child Have?

The type of angioedema a patient has is most easily determined by their symptoms, although a medical diagnosis is essential.

Types of Angioedema

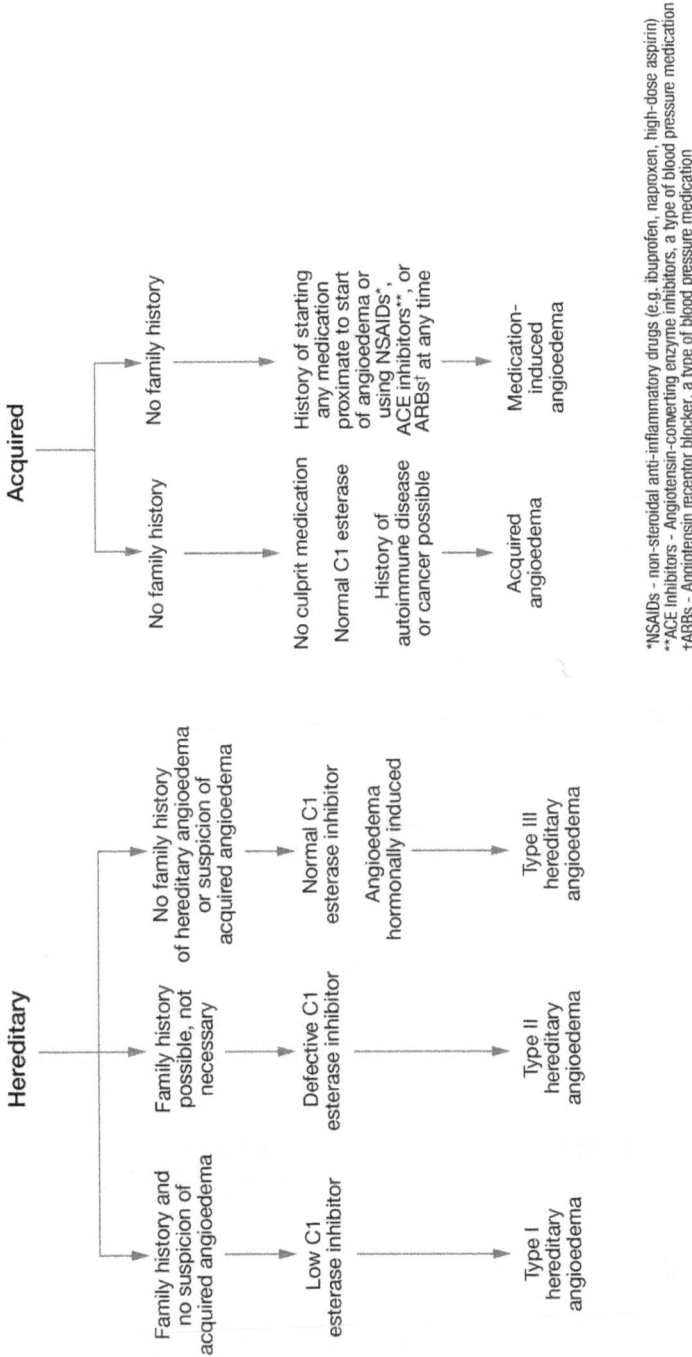

Hereditary

- Family history and no suspicion of acquired angioedema → Low C1 esterase inhibitor → Type I hereditary angioedema
- Family history possible, not necessary → Defective C1 esterase inhibitor → Type II hereditary angioedema
- No family history of hereditary angioedema or suspicion of acquired angioedema → Normal C1 esterase inhibitor → Angioedema hormonally induced → Type III hereditary angioedema

Acquired

- No family history → No culprit medication / Normal C1 esterase / History of autoimmune disease or cancer possible → Acquired angioedema
- No family history → History of starting any medication proximate to start of angioedema or using NSAIDs*, ACE inhibitors**, or ARBs† at any time → Medication-induced angioedema

*NSAIDs - non-steroidal anti-inflammatory drugs (e.g. ibuprofen, naproxen, high-dose aspirin)
**ACE inhibitors - Angiotensin-converting enzyme inhibitors, a type of blood pressure medication
†ARBs - Angiotensin receptor blocker, a type of blood pressure medication

Figure 27: Diagnosis and treatment of the various types of angioedema.

Hereditary angioedema - If there is a family history of idiopathic angioedema, or the swelling occurs randomly but also occurs after trauma (such as a car wreck) or after surgery and the usual medications do not work, it is likely due to the enzyme deficiency of C1 esterase. If it is hormone related in nature, it is most likely due to Type III HAE or Factor 12 abnormality.

Acquired angioedema - If there is no clear pattern, the angioedema started after a virus or infection, around the same time as another autoimmune disease or cancer was diagnosed, or during a period of extreme stress, it is an autoimmune type of angioedema that is said to be acquired.

Medication-induced angioedema - If the angioedema begins any time after starting one of the drugs implicated as causative, it is likely medication-induced from NSAIDs or opioid-analgesics, ACE inhibitors, or ARBs (or at least it is worth a several-month trial of the patient going off of that medication).

Allergic angioedema from other medication - If it starts within a short period of time after any other medication, it is likely allergic angioedema from that medication.

Allergic urticaria - If the angioedema symptoms come and go in response to a specific exposure, it is likely allergic urticaria. When the urticaria is located in areas of thin skin and subcutaneous tissue like the face, hands, and feet, or if the hives are particularly large, they may resemble the generalized swelling of angioedema instead of discrete hives.

Occasionally, if we are uncertain that the rash is angioedema, we may request a skin biopsy. We may also request additional tests if we mutually decide to start certain medications (see Medications for Allergic Angioedema Flares below).

NOTE
Only allergic angioedema is triggered by an allergy

The only form of angioedema caused by allergies is allergic angioedema. The other forms of angioedema, whether they are caused by NSAIDs, ACE-inhibitors, hereditary angioedema due to C1 esterase deficiency or disfunction, or Type III hereditary angioedema due to hormonal events, even though they resemble allergic angioedema perfectly, they are NOT caused by allergies. This is because the end result is caused by the same mediators (bradykinin) as those of allergic angioedema. The triggers and the cause differentiate the types of angioedema.

Medications for Allergic Angioedema Flares

For allergic angioedema, since histamines and leukotrienes are released from allergic cells when your child is having a flare-up, antihistamines like Benadryl and anti-leukotrienes are used to control the symptoms.

Anti-H1 Histamines

We have medications for two of the four known histamine receptors. Below is a list of common antihistamines for the H1 receptor (see Table 2). Their primary side effects are dryness of the eyes, mouth, and skin, reflux symptoms or gastrointestinal discomfort, and sedation. Also, antihistamines should only be taken according to your child's allergist's instruction, and they should not be taken with some common antibiotics, as the combination may cause a heart rhythm disturbance which can be fatal, albeit rarely. Allergic reaction is always a potential side effect of all medications, although it is rare.

Table 2

Anti-H1 Histamines		Time to response	Time to relapse	Potential for remission
Medication				
Age	Dose			
Loratadine+ (Claritin or Alavert)		Several days	Several days	No. Not satisfactory in up to 50% of patients
2 to <6 years**	2.5 mg 1 time/day			
6 to <12 years**	5 mg 1 time/day			
12 years to adult	10 mg 1 time/day			
Fexofenadine+ (Allegra)		Same	Same	No
6 to <12 years**	30 mg every 12 hours to max 60 mg/day			
12 years to adult	60 mg every 12 hours to max 120 mg/day			
Adults	60 mg every 12 hours to max 180 mg/day			
Cetirizine*+ (Zyrtec)		Same	Same	No
2 to <6 years**	2.5-5 mg 1 time/day			
6 to <12 years**	5-10 mg 1 time/day			
12 years to adult	10 mg 1 time/day			
Levocetirizine*+ (Xyzal)		Same	Same	No
2 to <6 years**	1.25 mg 1 time/day			
6 to <12 years**	2.5 mg 1 time/day			
12 years to adult	2.5-5 mg 1 time/day			
Cyproheptadine* (Periactin)		Same	Same	No
Up to <2 years**	Consult Physician			
2 to 6 years**	2 mg 2-3 times/day to max 12 mg/day			
7 to 14 years	4 mg 2-4 times/day to max 16 mg/day			
14 years to adult	0.5 mg/kg 1 time/day to max 32 mg/day			
Doxepin* (Sinequan)		Same	Same	No
<12 years**	Not advised			
Adults only	75 mg 2-4 times/day to max 300 mg			
Hydroxyzine* (Atarax, Vistaril)**		Same	Same	No
To <6 years**	Consult Physician			
6 to <12 years**	12.5-25 mg 4 times/day to max 50-100 mg/day			
12 years to adult	25-100 mg 4 times/day to max 400 mg/day			

*Can be sedating. Test at bedtime before using during the day. If it is sedating, restrict to bedtime and do not take with other sedating drugs like alcohol, codeine, etc.
**Consult with your physician before giving medication to any child age six and under.
+Over-the-counter

Claritin, Alavert, Allegra, Zyrtec, Xyzal, Periactin, Sinequan, Atarax, Vistaril. Full prescribing information. Various manufacturers; 2022.

Anti-H2 Histamines

The second type of antihistamine (H2) medications listed below are most commonly used for indigestion and all are now available over-the-counter. Use according to your child's allergist-immunologist's directions and doses, manufacturer's recommendations, and with their attendant precautions.

Table 3

Anti-H2 Histamines				
Medication		Time to response	Potential for remission	Monitoring
Age	Dose			
Cimetidine+ (Tagamet)		15 minutes to several days	None	None
<12 years >12 years Adults	Consult Physician 30-40 mg/kg per day divided in 4 doses 400-800 mg 2 times/day			
Famotidine+ (Pepcid)		Same	None	None
<12 years >12 years Adults	Consult Physician 1 mg/kg per day divided in 2 doses 20 mg 2 times/day			
Nizatidine+ (Axid)		Same	None	None
<12 years >12 years Adult	Consult Physician 10 mg/kg per day divided in 2 doses 150 mg 2 times/day or 300 mg 1 time/day at bedtime			

+Over-the-counter
Tagamet, Pepcid, Axid. Full prescribing information. Various manufacturers; 2022.

Table 4

Anti-Leukotrienes				
Medication		Time to Response	Time to Relapse	Potential for Remission
Age	Dose			
Montelukast (Singulair)				
2 to 5 years 6 to 14 years 12 years to adult	4 mg per day 5 mg per day 10 mg per day	Several days to 1 week	Several days	+/-
Zileuton CR (Zyflo CR)				
12 years to adult	1200 mg 2 times/day	Several days to 1 week	Several days	+/-
Zafirlukast (Accolate)				
5 to <12 years 12 years to adult	10 mg 2 times/day 20 mg 2 times/day	Several days to 1 week	Several days	+/-

Singulair, Zyflo CR, Accolate. Full prescribing information. Various manufacturers; 2022.

Anti-Leukotrienes

Anti-leukotrienes block chemicals that provoke symptoms similar to histamines, but because they use different receptors, different medications are needed. Following is a list of anti-leukotrienes.

Table 3 continued

Adverse effects
Common: Headache abdominal pain, dizziness, diarrhea, somnolence. Rare to very rare: Nausea, vomiting, constipation, mood changes, weakness, muscle cramps, joint pain, insomnia, dry mouth, allergic reaction including liver and kidney damage and drug interactions, bloody and black tarry stools, clay colored stools, irregular pulse and palpitations, confusion, hallucinations, memory problems, trouble breathing, trouble urinating (and in adults, sexual dysfunction), major blood issues. Unique to cimetidine: interferes with other drugs that use same liver enzyme.
Same
Same Low levels of NDMA found in these products

Table 4 continued

Adverse Effects	Monitoring
Headache Gastrointestinal complaints Mood changes Night terrors Allergic reaction	None
Same; liver and bleeding problems if not stopped when liver damage a problem (see monitoring); drug interactions; allergic reaction	Baseline: Liver enzymes and prothrombin time. Monthly for 3 months, then every 3 months for 1 year, then annually, then periodically.
Same; liver and bleeding problems if not stopped when liver damage a problem (see monitoring); drug interactions; allergic reaction	Baseline: Liver enzymes, prothrombin time. Monthly for 3 months, then every 3 months for 1 year, then for 1 year, then periodically.

Table 5

Treatment of Hereditary Angioedema, Side Effects, and Recommendations for Use

Medication	Mechanism	Route	Onset
C1-esterase inhibitor (Berinert)	Plasma-derived C1-esterase inhibitor (replaces deficient or defective protein)	IV	15 minutes
C1-esterase inhibitor (Cinryze)	Plasma-derived C1-esterase inhibitor (replaces deficient or defective protein)	IV	60 minutes
Icatabant (Firazyr)	Bradykinin B2 receptor antagonist	SC	45 minutes to reach peak levels, 2-2.5 hours to stop an attack
C1-esterase inhibitor (Haegarda)	Plasma-derived C1-esterase inhibitor (replaces deficient or defective protein)	SC	Most issues resolved within 1 day of treatment initiation
Icatabant (generic)	Bradykinin B2 receptor antagonist	SC	Median time of onset of symptom relief is 2 hours
Ecallantide (Kalbitor)	Plasma kallikrein inhibitor	SC	Significant decrease in symptoms of attack within 4 hours of injection
Berotralstat (Orladeyo)	Plasma kallikrein inhibitor	Oral	Between 6-12 days
C1-esterase inhibitor (Ruconest)	Plasma-derived C1-esterase inhibitor (replaces deficient or defective protein)	IV	Eases symptoms in an average of 75 minutes
Lanadelumab-flyo (Takhzyro)	Monoclonal antibody kallikrein inhibitor	SC	May work immediately; takes up to 70 days to be at steady level

Terminology used in this table
IV – intravenous
SC – subcutaneous

Indicated for Ages	Quick Onset v. Prevention	Common Side Effects	Comments
Pediatric and adult (studied down to 5 years old)	Quick Onset	Allergic reaction, arterial and venous thromboembolic events (clots), ability to transmit infectious agents from blood (it is a blood product) such as viruses and, hypothetically, prions. Plus taste disorder in 4%, worsening of angioedema attacks, headache, abdominal pain and discomfort, rash, nasopharyngitis, nausea, vulvovaginal mycotic infection, influenza-like illness, and upper respiratory tract infection	There is not enough information to assess risk in the very young, very old, during pregnancy or lactation
6 years and older	Prevention	Same as above. Plus rash, itching, headache, vomiting, fever, catheter site pain, redness, dizziness	Same as above
18 years and older	Quick Onset	Injection site reactions, fever, liver function enzyme elevations, dizziness, rash	Same as above
6 years and older	Quick Onset	Same as above (Berinert). Plus injection site reaction, nasopharyngitis, dizziness	Same as above
18 years and older	Quick Onset	Injection site reactions, fever, liver function enzyme elevations, dizziness, rash	Same as above
12 years and older	Quick Onset	Allergic reaction and anaphylaxis; headache, nausea, vomiting, diarrhea, fever, injection site reactions, nasopharyngitis, itching, rash, hives, abdominal pain	Administered by a health professional Same as above
12 years and older	Prevention	Abdominal pain, vomiting, diarrhea, back pain and GERD; may promote abnormal heart rhythms if used in higher than recommended doses or in combination with certain drugs; headache, fatigue, rash, flatulence, elevations in liver enzymes	Same as above
2 years and older	Quick Onset	Allergic reaction, arterial and venous thromboembolic events (clots), headache nausea and diarrhea, sneezing, worsening angioedema, erythema marginatum, skin burning sensation, back pain, C-reactive protein increase, Fibrin D-dimer increase, lipoma, and vertigo	Same as above
12 years and older	Prevention	Allergic reaction, injection site reactions, upper respiratory infections, headache, rash, myalgia, dizziness, and diarrhea, myalgia, liver enzyme elevations	Same as above

Berinert, Cinryze, Firazyr, Haegarda, Icatabant (generic), Kalbitor, Orladeyo, Ruconest. Full prescribing information. Various manufacturers; 2022.

Chemotherapy for Angioedema

These medications are stronger drugs designed to suppress the immune system. As a result, they have more side effects and are not for everyone. Masking the symptoms with antihistamines and anti-leukotrienes never solves the actual problem and, for acquired angioedema, is frequently insufficient. Many patients need to take milder forms of chemotherapy to put them in remission from angioedema.

Corticosteroids

Corticosteroids, like prednisone, are commonly prescribed for angioedema. These work very rapidly and are known to help, but may not be sufficient to put your child's angioedema in remission. Using them frequently or in high doses can be problematic due to the many side effects, which include but are not limited to problems with the bones, joints, muscles, sugar control, blood pressure, and cholesterol control. In addition, your child's own adrenal glands make corticosteroids daily and these help control many essential metabolic processes. They are suppressed when you take systemic corticosteroids and can stop working permanently, making them steroid-dependent or causing death. Therefore, it is best to avoid use of systemic corticosteroids except when throat closure or airway compromise occurs.

Medications for Hereditary Angioedema

Hereditary angioedema, as previously explained, is caused by a C1 esterase deficiency. Antihistamines, anti-leukotrienes, corticosteroids, and epinephrine pens do not work like they do in response to allergic angioedema because hereditary angioedema is not caused by an allergic reaction.

For C1 esterase deficiency, the medications in Table 5 either replace C1 esterase or disrupt the symptoms of increased vascular permeability and inflammation.

Treatment for Drug-Induced Angioedema

The best treatment for angioedema caused by a drug—whether allergic angioedema or the result of chemical inhibition—is to avoid the trigger drug.

Chapter 9

Breathe Free: Therapeutic Strategies to Reduce Asthma Severity

Chapter Preview

- What is asthma and what are its most concerning symptoms?
- What are the steps in diagnosing asthma and its severity?
- Which therapeutic strategies are being used successfully to reduce the severity of asthma attacks?
- How preventing allergies can stop the development of asthma.
- The risks and benefits of medications prescribed for asthma.

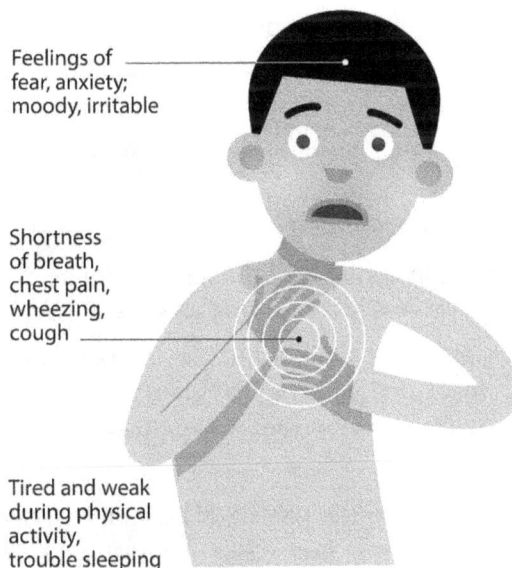

Feelings of fear, anxiety; moody, irritable

Shortness of breath, chest pain, wheezing, cough

Tired and weak during physical activity, trouble sleeping

Figure 28: Symptoms of an asthma attack.

What Is Asthma?

Asthma is a serious chronic lung disease causing inflammation of the lungs characterized by intermittent or persistent shortness of breath, wheezing, chest tightness, and/or cough. These symptoms worsen in the presence of triggers, which are unique to each patient.

If you have asthma, you are not alone. According to the Centers for Disease Control and Prevention (CDC), over 25 million people in the United States (or 7.8% of the population) have been told they have asthma at some point in their lifetime. This number has been steadily increasing—since 2001, almost 5 million additional people have been diagnosed with asthma. In my state of Arizona, over 500,000 people (9.6% of the population) had asthma in 2020 (CDC 2022). This is fairly representative of most states. Diagnosis rate and differences in populations across the country may account for some differences.

Medical Care Needed by Asthmatic Patients

Over 10 million patients with asthma (41%) had one or more asthma attacks within the previous 12 months (2019); 42.7% were children and 40.7% were adults. Almost 170,000 were hospitalized for asthma in 2018: 64,525 children and 104,805 adults. Asthma patients made over 10.5 million doctor visits in 2018 and over 1.8 million emergency department visits in 2019.

As you can imagine, the cost of asthma is enormous. From 2002-2007, the total estimated cost of asthma in the United States was $56 billion: $50.1 billion direct health care costs and $5.9 billion indirect costs, such as lost productivity at work. In 2013, the estimated direct and indirect costs of asthma ballooned to $81.9 billion (Nurgmagambetov 2017). The United States is expected to spend over $300 billion of direct costs associated with asthma through 2038 (Yaghoubi 2019).

Asthma Can Be Life-Threatening

An important consideration in caring for yourself or a loved one with a diagnosis of asthma is that over 4,000 deaths from asthma occurred in 2019 in the U.S. Of them, 1,682 were male; 2,463 were female. Further, deaths occurred in all age ranges: 16 were 0-4 years old; 91 were 5-11 years old; 97 were 12-17 years old; 158 were 18-24 years old; 348 were 24-34 years old; 1,725 were 35-64 years old; and 1,710 were 65+ years old.

In 2020, after trending down between 2001-2009, the number of deaths from asthma increased to 4,145, or 12.6 deaths per one million people in the population.

Eighty-seven of these deaths were in Arizona, claiming 11.7 lives per million people in the state's population. When one considers that we live in a developed country, these statistics are sobering.

PATHOLOGY OF ASTHMA

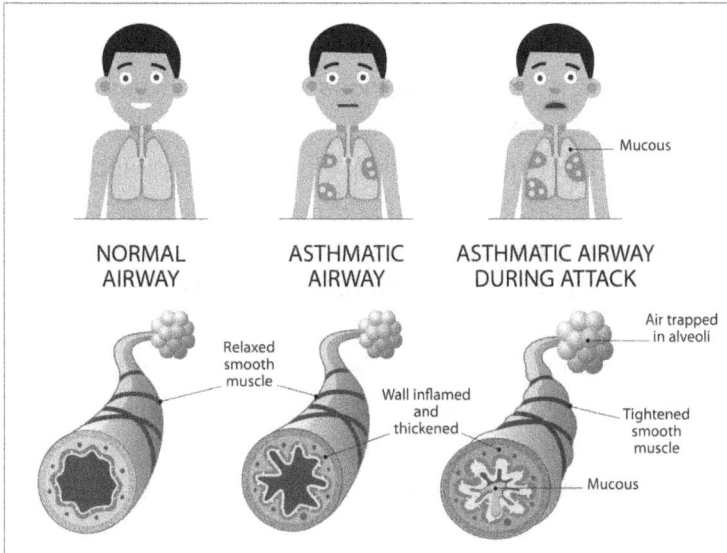

Figure 29: The normal bronchioles—tube-like passages through which air enters and leaves the lung during breathing—are wide open and the smooth muscle that surrounds them is relaxed. During an asthma attack, that smooth muscle surrounding the bronchiole tubes constricts, the walls of the tubes become inflamed and thickened, and mucous fills these tubes. Together, this causes decreased diameter through which air can flow and trapping of air in the alveoli, the cells through which gas exchange occurs. This results in shortness of breath, wheezing, chest tightness, and excess mucous production.

Understanding Asthma

There are three hallmarks of an asthmatic lung: inflammation, mucous production, and bronchoconstriction.

Inflammation causes irritation, swelling, and thickening of the airway wall. These changes can be temporary and result in decreased ability of the airway to exchange oxygen and move air normally. Inflammation refers to the many cells that are found in the lung as a result of poorly-controlled asthma. This drives and perpetuates the process.

Mucous is produced by glands in the airway. It can cause coughing and may plug the airway, making breathing even more difficult.

Bronchoconstriction is caused by the tightening of the muscles that encircle the bronchial tubes. It decreases the diameter of the asthmatic airway and affects the ability of the lungs to exhale old air out and inhale fresh air. The combined effects of the inflamed and thickened airway wall, mucous in the airway, and bronchoconstriction cause difficulty in taking a breath.

Over time this process may be less reversible as a result of chronic inflammation; at that point, the "quick rescue" drugs are less likely to resolve the issue.

Bronchodilators are drugs that relax the muscle of the bronchioles (or "air tubes") of the lung, increasing the diameter of those air tubes and easing the ability of the asthma patient to take a breath. They may make asthma patients feel better quickly and temporarily ease bronchoconstriction. However, bronchodilators do not affect inflammation or mucous production. Therefore, when the temporary relief of bronchoconstriction wears off, patients are in as bad or worse condition than before the bronchodilator was used. This is why bronchodilators like Albuterol are called "rescue" drugs.

Bronchodilators are not a maintenance drug; they have no impact on the overall disease process of asthma. While some patients only use a rescue medication occasionally, any patient who is overusing it should also have a daily maintenance medication that targets the inflammation and mucous production.

What Causes Asthma?

Asthma is caused by a combination of environmental, genetic, and lifestyle factors. Exposure to childhood respiratory illnesses and allergens may increase the risk of asthma. On the other hand, exposure to many different animals may decrease the risk of asthma. The genetics of asthma are complicated, but multiple genes have been identified and linked with asthma, some for increased risk and others for increased protection from the disease. Obesity and a sedentary lifestyle also increase the risk and severity of asthma. To summarize, there is no way to predict with certainty and no one test that is going to predict whether your wheezing child will go on to have asthma.

Of course, concerned parents want to know the risk of their child having asthma in later life. Currently, the most-used prediction strategy is the Asthma Predictive Indices (API), which evaluate the risk of asthma diagnosis in the future for children aged three or less who suffer from recurrent wheezing. The two different APIs look at slightly different aspects to estimate the likelihood of whether a child will develop asthma in later life. This is an educated guess, not an absolute.

Predictive Value of the API - Stringent Index

Criteria for a positive stringent index includes frequent wheezing during a child's first three years plus one major risk factor (parental history of asthma or eczema), or two of three minor risk factors (high eosinophil white blood count, wheezing without colds, and allergic rhinitis). Either combination of risk factors portends a 76% rate of active asthma by age five or six.

Over 95% of children with a negative stringent index never had active asthma between ages six and thirteen (Castro-Rodriguez 2000).

Predictive Value of the API - Loose Index

A loose index requires any wheeze at all under the age of three years old plus the other risk factors listed above. Of those children with a positive loose index, 59% will go on to develop asthma by school age (Castro-Rodriguez 2000).

Allergy Shots Can Interrupt the Development of Asthma and Decrease Its Severity

Can anything reduce the risk of developing allergic asthma long-term? The only treatment we have found that can significantly reduce this risk is allergy shots. I highly recommend them to my young patients. Aggressively addressing and treating every condition and trigger that exacerbates asthma is, in my experience, a very effective way of controlling asthma.

I have worked with many young children who have terrible asthma and frequent flares. But once we tame their top trigger—environmental allergies—with asthma shots, most are able to reduce their medication and no longer have the unpredictable, disabling, and frightening attacks that send them to the emergency department and damage their lungs. For this reason, it is very important you see a board-certified allergist-immunologist as early as possible if you think your child may have asthma.

I also have a working theory that, in general, aggressive treatment during youth prevents progression of asthma. Early in my career, I saw many young patients in their 20s and 30s who had asthma as children and had already developed chronic obstructive pulmonary disease (COPD). This means they had long-term damage to their airway, so their quick-acting rescue bronchodilators like albuterol no longer worked. Decades later, my young patients with the same type of severe asthma seem to be much more likely to go into remission when they are young adults due to the combination of early, aggressive treatment and better medications and biologics.

Because early use of allergy shots prevents progression to other allergic diseases and asthma, it is widely held that the earlier the treatment, the better. Also, working with a board-certified allergist-immunologist who understands all of the tools at their disposal and is more likely to aggressively treat the patient is a distinct advantage.

Controlling Environmental Allergies May Also Help Children Avoid Developing Asthma

Children diagnosed with atopic dermatitis and sensitivity to air-borne allergens are at greater risk for developing asthma with these risk factors. However, population studies suggest that allergy shots can prevent progression to asthma when given early in life (recall that allergic rhinitis is also a minor risk factor in developing asthma) (Gradman 2021). Also, use of skin barrier protection techniques like moisturization can prevent accumulation of additional allergies in patients with eczema and in so doing, can prevent development of asthma (Khani 2018; Kaper 2018; Kim 2018; Myers 2010).

Food Allergies and Asthma

Food can be a major trigger for asthma attacks in many children with asthma. The most common asthma triggers are the same as those that cause allergic reactions: egg, wheat, soy, milk, peanut, tree nuts, fish, shellfish, and sesame. However, even children without asthma can experience some of the symptoms generally attributed to asthma, such as chest tightness, wheezing, and shortness of breath, during a major allergic reaction. This does not mean those children have asthma. However, some of the dysfunctional processes behind both issues can be similar and therefore have some symptoms in common.

Diagnosis of Asthma Requires Evaluating Airway Volumes

Asthma is diagnosed with a detailed medical history, physical examination, and either spirometry or pulmonary function testing that shows a partially reversible airflow obstruction (i.e., difficulty blowing air out of the lungs that can be partially normalized with a bronchodilator like albuterol). Asthma is characterized by some or all of these recurrent symptoms: shortness of breath, wheezing, chest tightness, and/or cough that worsens with certain triggers. Sometimes other tests are required to definitively diagnose asthma and to rule out other conditions.

Assessing airway volume and function is critical to understanding asthma severity in adults and children old enough to perform spirometry or pulmonary function testing. Essentially, large and small airway volumes are estimated and compared to populations of a similar age, weight, size, and ethnicity. A decrease in the large or small airway is known as an obstruction, meaning the patient has difficulty exhaling gas from their lungs. When the exhalation volume can be increased after administration of a bronchodilator, the lung issue is then considered to be reversible.

Another test I use to aid in diagnosing my patients is The Childhood Asthma Control Test™ (C-ACT) which has been validated as a test of asthma control (Schatz 2006; Liu 2010). A score of 19 or less on the C-ACT identifies children with the lowest level of control.

According to the GINA guidelines, your child's asthma may be uncontrolled if they:

- Have two or more asthma attacks per year requiring systemic steroids;
- Wake up two or more nights per month with symptoms of asthma; and/or
- Have wheezing, chest tightness, cough, or shortness of breath two or more times per week.

According to the National Heart, Lung, and Blood Institute (NHLBI), knowing the frequency of your child's asthma symptoms enables the allergist-immunologist to classify the severity of their asthma as mild, moderate, or severe, with further classification as intermittent or persistent. This classification matrix guides recommended medications and interventions (see Table 6 and Table 7).

In order to determine the patient's grade of asthma, the allergist-immunologist classifies the asthma as intermittent or persistent, and subclassifies persistent as mild, moderate, or severe. This is important, as treatment is based on the frequency and severity of symptoms and on the ability of short-acting bronchodilators to control symptoms.

Key to scoring the C-ACT Test

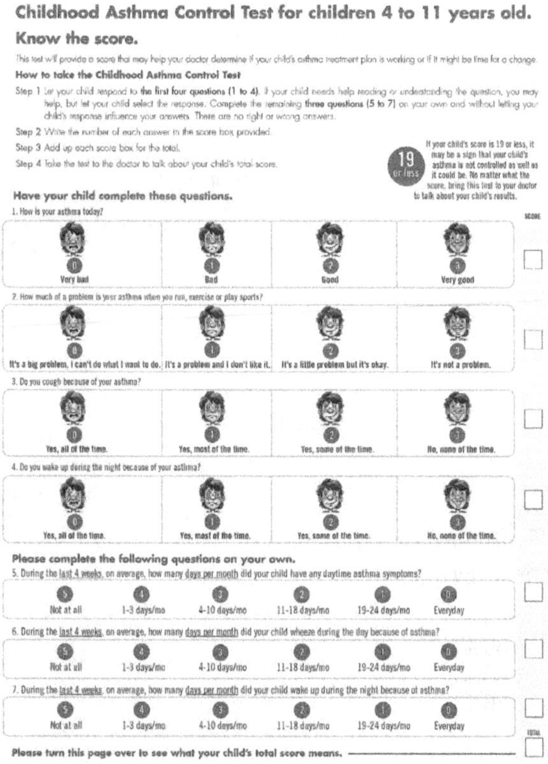

Figure 30: Childhood Asthma Control Test (C-ACT)

Figure 31: Key to Childhood Asthma Control Test (C-ACT)

Table 6

Classification of Asthma Severity and Recommendations for Treatment

Components of Severity		Intermittent	
Impairment	Frequency of Symptoms	≤2 days/week	
	Nighttime Awakenings	**Age**	**Frequency**
		0 to 4 years	None
		≥5 years	≤2 times/mo.
	Rescue Meds Used for Symptom Control (short-acting Beta2-agonist)	≤2 days/week	
	Interference with Normal Activity	None	
	Lung Function Testing >5 years old	• Normal FEV1 between exacerbations • FEV1 > 80% predicted • FEV1/FVC Normal	
Risk	Exacerbations Requiring Systemic Corticosteroids	**Age**	**Frequency**
		0 to 4 years	0-1 time/year
		≥5 years	0-1 time/year

Normal Lung Function Test by Age	
Age	**Normal FEV1/FVC**
8 to 19 years	>85%
20 to 39 years	>80%
40 to 59 years	>80%
60 to 80 years	>70%

Classification of Asthma Severity					
Persistent					
Mild		Moderate		Severe	
>2 days/week, but not daily		Daily		Throughout the day	
Age	Frequency	Age	Frequency	Age	Frequency
0 to 4 years ≥5 years	1-2 times/mo. 3-4 times/mo.	0 to 4 years ≥5 years	3-4 times/mo. >1 time/week but not nightly	0 to 4 years ≥5 years	>1 time/week >1 time/week, nightly
3 to 6 days/week but less than 1 time/day		Daily		Several times/day	
Minor limitation		Some limitation		Extreme limitation	

• FEV1 >60% but
  < 80% predicted
• FEV1/FVC reduced
  by 5% predicted
		• FEV1 >60% but
		  < 80% predicted
		• FEV1/FVC reduced
		  by 5% predicted
				• FEV1 <60% predicted
				• FEV1/FVC reduced
				  by >5% predicted	

Age	Frequency
0 to 4 years	≥2 flares in 6 months requiring systemic steroids, or ≥4 wheezing episodes/year lasting >1 day and attributes of persistent asthma, or >2 flares/year.
≥5 years	≥2 flares/year

FEV1 = Forced expiratory volume in one second; the majority of lung volume is exhaled during this time.
FVC = Forced vital capacity is the total volume of air that can be exhaled from the lungs during best effort attempts.
FEV1/FVC = Ratio of forced expiratory volume in one second over the forced vital capacity; shows the ability of the lungs to move air. The greater the percentage, the better.

Table 7

Classification of Asthma Severity and Recommendations for Treatment (cont.)	
Recommendations for Asthma Treatment	
Intermittent Symptoms	
Age	Medication
0 to 4 years	Short-acting Beta agonist
5 to 11 years	Short-acting Beta agonist
≥6 years	Same as above
≥12 years	As needed low-dose ICS-formoterol or low-dose ICS with short-acting bronchodilator

*Terminology used in this table
ICS – Inhaled corticosteroids
LABA – Long-acting beta agonists or bronchodilators
LTRA – Leukotriene receptor antagonist
LTA – Leukotriene antagonist

| Recommendations for Asthma Treatment | | |
| Persistent Symptoms | | |
Mild	Moderate	Severe
Low dose ICS* Alternatives are cromolyn or montelukast	Medium-dose ICS and consider short course systemic corticosteroids for flares	Medium-dose ICS and consider short course systemic corticosteroids for flares; consider step up (addition of LABA or montelukast; increase to high-dose ICS)
Low dose ICS Alternatives are cromolyn, LTRA*, nedocromil, theophylline	Medium-dose ICS and either LABA* or montelukast; consider short course systemic corticosteroids for flares	As above; other alternatives include adding LTRA or theophylline; consider step up to high-dose ICS plus LABA +/- LTA* or theophylline +/- systemic oral steroids
Same as above	Same as above	As above; other alternatives +/- Anti-IgE, anti-IL5, anti-IL4/-13
Low dose ICS Alternatives are cromolyn, LTRA, nedocromil, theophylline	ICS and either LABA or montelukast; consider short course systemic corticosteroids for flares; alternatives are low dose ICS and either LTRA, theophylline or zileuton	As above; other alternatives Anti-IL5R

Adapted from the following resources:
National Institutes of Health. Managing asthma long term in children 0-4 years of age and 5-11 years of age. National Heart, Blood and Lung Institute website. Updated August 27, 2007. Accessed December 1, 2022. https://www.nhlbi.nih.gov/files/docs/guidelines/08_sec4_lt_0-11.pdf
National Institutes of Health. Focused updates to the asthma management guidelines: A report from the National Asthma Education and Prevention Program Coordinating Committee Expert Panel Working Group. National Heart, Blood and Lung Institute website. Updated February, 2021. Accessed November 20, 2022. https://www.nhlbi.nih.gov/resources/2020-focused-updates-asthma-management-guidelines.

ASTHMA
SYMPTOMS

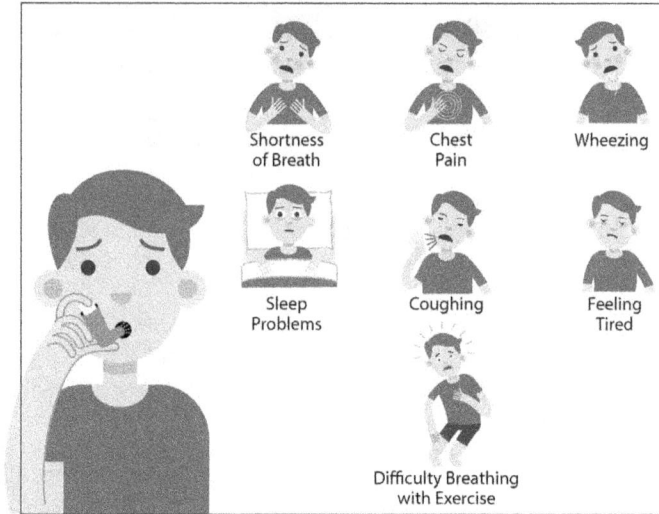

ASTHMA
TRIGGERS

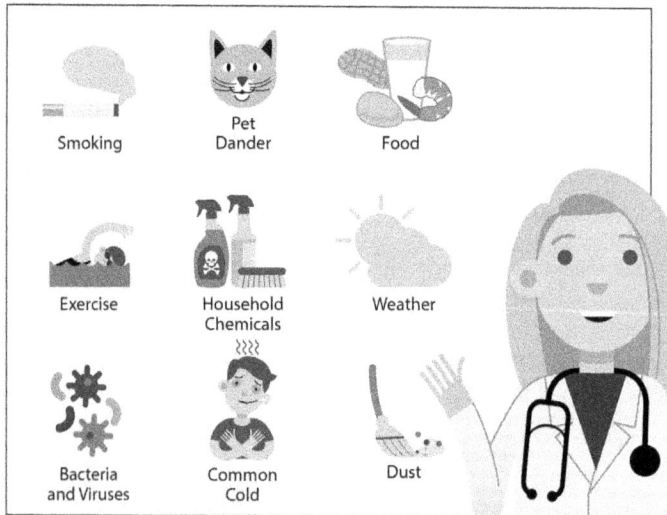

Figure 32: Asthma symptoms and triggers

Identify Your Asthma Triggers

After classifying the patient's asthma severity, the next step is to identify and avoid the triggers that cause their flares. Typical triggers are foods and/or food additives, exercise, lung and other infections, stress, allergic inhalants (such as mold spores, pollen, pet dander, dust mites, and/or cockroach parts), irritants (such as chemicals and smoke), changes in weather and temperature, strong emotion and stress, medications, vocal cord dysfunction, acid reflux, and hormonal changes.

If You Can't Avoid Triggers

Your triggers should be avoided whenever possible. If avoidance is not possible, eliminating them with allergy immunotherapy—allergy shots—is ideal (Fritzsching 2021; Penagos 2022).

Premedication is another effective way to reduce the severity of an asthmatic reaction. Using a rescue inhaler 20 minutes before exercise is just one example of the way changing medication timing, dose, and/or frequency can help.

Weighing the Risks and Rewards of Adding Maintenance Medication

Maintenance medication involves an inhaled steroid that decreases the ongoing inflammation at the root of asthma and asthma flares. Many mothers and patients are nervous about using these medications regularly because they contain steroids, and they're concerned about the possible side-effects those steroids may have.

Their concern is understandable. My approach is to prescribe only the amount of medication needed and to constantly re-evaluate the patient's response to their medications so we can decrease their intake when possible. This is one reason why I like to see young asthma patients every three months.

At the same time, as I mentioned before, it is my experience that aggressively treating young children tends to *decrease* symptoms and avoid damage to their lungs in the long run.

Also, if you hold back the maintenance medication but your child has severe flares that require systemic steroids, you have not really decreased their risk of medication side effects, but have unintentionally increased it. Just one course of systemic steroids has the metabolic effect of taking the most potent inhaled steroid *for five years*. To explain, while you do get some minimal systemic exposure with inhaled steroid maintenance medication, the overwhelming majority of those steroids are directed at the lungs where we want and need it. However, in an emergency, we have to use much higher doses of systemic steroids to get the amount we need to the lung.

Long story short: If your child was prescribed a maintenance medication, have them use it exactly as directed and return to your allergist-immunologist every three months to reassess. At that time, the dose and frequency may be adjusted because the child may not need the medication all year around or need the same amount all year.

Try to keep in mind these medications are not prescribed as an easy fix. Your frequent visits to assess how well the medications are controlling their symptoms are also my opportunity to monitor the potential side-effects, as detailed in the table below.

Table 8

Asthma Medications, Side Effects, and Recommendations for Use

Rescue Medication for Symptom Relief

Medication	Mechanism
Short-acting bronchodilator (albuterol sulfate)	Activates beta2 receptors on bronchial smooth muscle, relaxing airway and opening airway temporarily
Inhaled corticosteroids-ICS (formoterol)	ICS reduces inflammation; formoterol relaxes bronchial smooth muscle, opening airway

Prevention & Control Medication for Symptom Control

Medication	Mechanism
ICS (budesonide, ciclesonide, fluticasone, beclomethasone, mometasone)	ICS reduces inflammation
ICS-LABA* Inhaled corticosteroids–long-acting Beta agonists (mometasone-formoterol, fluticasone-salmeterol, budesonide-formoterol)	ICS reduces inflammation; formoterol relaxes bronchial smooth muscle, opening airway
Systemic corticosteroids (prednisone, dexamethasone, methylprednisolone)	Systemic anti-inflammatory effects
LAMA Long-acting muscarinic inhalers (tiotropium)	Causes bronchodilation and opens airway
ICS-LABA-LAMA* (fluticasone furoate-umeclidinium-vilanterol)	ICS reduces inflammation; LABA relaxes bronchial smooth muscle, opening airway; LAMA causes bronchodilation and opens airway
Anti-IgE (omalizumab)	Inhibits binding of IgE to IgE receptors on allergic cells, decreasing release of mediators of allergy
Anti-IL-5 (mepolizumab)	Prevents activation of immune cells that contribute to asthma
Anti-IL-5 (reslizumab)	Prevents activation of immune cells that contribute to asthma
Anti-IL5R-alpha (benrilizumab)	Decreases number of immune cells that contribute to asthma
Anti-IL4R-alpha (dupilumab)	Blocks IL-4 and IL-13, preventing allergic cells from turning "on"

*Terminology used in this table
ICS – Inhaled corticosteroids
LABA – Long-acting beta agonists or bronchodilators
LAMA - Long-acting muscarinic agonists

Common Side Effects	Comments
Rapid heart rate, cardiotoxicity, nervousness or shakiness, headache, throat or nasal irritation, and muscle aches, electrolyte disturbances, other irritation, sweating, seizures	If using excessively (twice per week unexpectedly, twice per month on awakening), return to physician for medication review
Thrush, upper respiratory tract infection, cough, throat irritation, headache	Gargle with water after use

Common Side Effects	Comments
Thrush, upper respiratory tract infection, cough, throat irritation, headache	Gargle with water after use
Thrush, upper respiratory tract infection, cough, throat irritation, headache	Gargle with water after use
Increased risk of fracture, infection, diabetes, hypertension, osteoporosis, obesity, increased appetite, adrenal suppression, and mood and behavior issues	Use lowest dose for shortest duration
Upper respiratory tract infection, cough, dry mouth, constipation	
Thrush, upper respiratory tract infection, cough, throat irritation, headache, dry mouth	
Local reaction, anaphylaxis, joint aches, general fatigue, dizziness	Administered under supervision of an experienced Allergist or Pulmonologist; black box warning for anaphylaxis; indicated for >6 years old
Local reaction, can reactivate zoster, rarely anaphylaxis	Administered under supervision of an experienced Allergist or Pulmonologist; indicated for >6 years old
Local reaction; anaphylaxis	Administered under supervision of an experienced Allergist or Pulmonologist; black box warning for anaphylaxis; indicated for >18 years old
Local reaction; anaphylaxis	Administered under supervision of an experienced Allergist or Pulmonologists; indicated for >12 years old
Local reaction; anaphylaxis; and increased allergic cells (hypereosinophilia)	Administered under supervision of an experienced Allergist or Pulmonologists; indicated for >6 years old

Short-acting bronchodilator, ICS, ICS-LABA, systemic corticosteroids, LAMA, ICS-LABA-LAMA, Anti-IgE, Anti-IL-5, Anti-IL5R-alpha. Full prescribing information. Various manufacturers; 2022.

Asthma Triggers Vary Depending on the Season

Asthmatic flares vary throughout the year. Some asthma symptoms that require maximum medication when pollen is abundant in the spring and fall can be well controlled with the lowest level of medication in the summer—or perhaps without any medication at all. That same patient may require maximum medication again when temperatures drop radically in the fall around Halloween. Not only do allergies affect asthma, but the weather itself and changes in weather can affect asthma.

Medical Treatment of Asthma

A stepwise approach is taken to treat asthma and use of step-up/step-down treatment strategy is common. Essentially, treatment is started and improvement assessed at regular intervals. If control is not adequate, treatment is increased—a step-up. If control is adequate after three to six months, the allergist-immunologist may attempt to reduce the medication dose and treatment frequency—a step down.

Other health conditions that may create or worsen an asthmatic flare need to be identified and remediated as a step in asthma care. These include sinusitis, rhinitis, acid reflux or GERD, obesity, obstructive sleep apnea, vocal cord dysfunction, depression, food allergies, and stress. Treating issues before they occur, such as vaccinating against influenza and pneumonia, can prevent asthmatic flares by protecting against a more severe case of influenza or pneumonia. (Vaccinations cannot prevent you from contracting disease, but they can lessen the severity and make it easier to tolerate.)

Asthma is a chronic, reversible obstructive airway disease and therefore needs to be reassessed regularly. It is especially important to re-assess young lungs regularly, as they are growing and developing.

Further, giving the patient some sense of control and empowerment is important. When a flare occurs, the patient may have to act on their own without treatment decisions from their doctor. This is why every asthma patient should have a customized Asthma Action Plan (see Asthma Action Plan in the Appendix).

Chapter 10

Hives: The Itch That is Skin Deep

Chapter Preview

- What are hives and what are the primary symptoms?
- How are hives related to allergies?
- Precautions about medications commonly prescribed for hives.

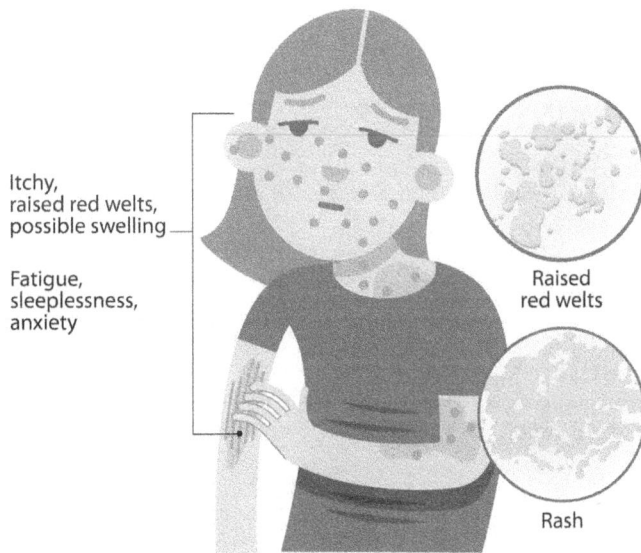

Itchy,
raised red welts,
possible swelling

Fatigue,
sleeplessness,
anxiety

Raised
red welts

Rash

Figure 33: Top symptoms of hives or urticaria.

What Are Hives?

Hives (or urticaria) is the name of a rash that looks like one or more mosquito bites all over the body. Just like mosquito bites, they can be swollen and red, intensely itchy or sometimes burning, and isolated or grouped together. The size can be as small as a pinpoint to very large. If they are big enough or in an area of the body where the subcutaneous tissue is smaller, like the face or hands, they may look more like swelling or angioedema. Hives can be the result of an allergy, an inherited condition, or an autoimmune disease. Allergies to a wide variety of substances can trigger hives, such as drugs; foods or food additives; inhalation, ingestion, or contact with allergic substances such as tree, grass, and weed pollen; dog, cat, and animal dander; mold spores; medications; and insects. Non-allergic triggers like scratching, vibration, heat, cold, sun, sweating, and pressure may initiate hives in patients with the autoimmune variety.

As with angioedema, the inherited and acquired autoimmune forms of hives are not the result of allergy and therefore are not easily tested. There is usually some form of autoimmune disease (thyroid disease, rheumatoid arthritis, vitiligo, etc.) noted in the patient or in a family member, although it may not be an immediate family member and is not necessary for diagnosis.

An autoimmune disease occurs when the immune system (the system of the body that protects you from infection) attacks itself with antibodies. Of course, antibodies are proteins meant to protect you from infection by sticking to bacteria- and virus-infected cells and flagging the immune system to rid your body of these potentially dangerous invaders.

AUTOIMMUNE FORM of CHRONIC HIVES

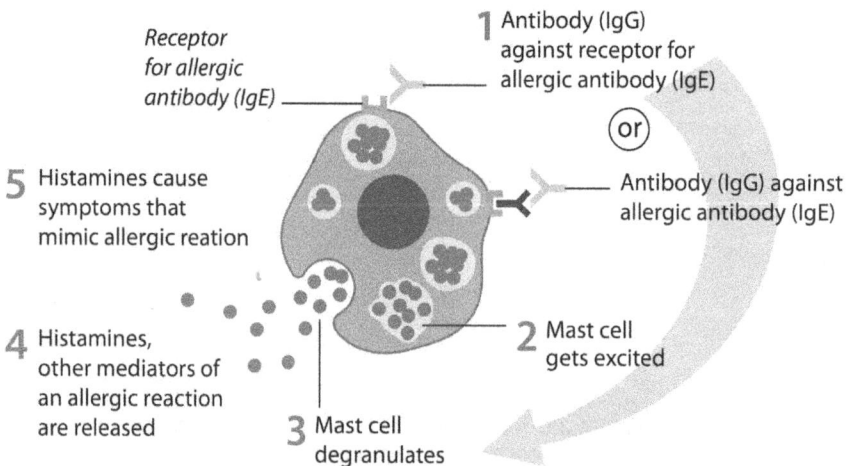

Receptor for allergic antibody (IgE)

1 Antibody (IgG) against receptor for allergic antibody (IgE)

(or)

Antibody (IgG) against allergic antibody (IgE)

5 Histamines cause symptoms that mimic allergic reation

4 Histamines, other mediators of an allergic reaction are released

2 Mast cell gets excited

3 Mast cell degranulates

Figure 34: Mast cell triggered by auto-immune antibodies, causing chronic hives. The most common causes of autoimmune hives result from IgG antibodies bound to the receptor for the antibody IgE (the allergic antibody) on mast cells or IgG to the allergic IgE flag. The IgG antibodies in step 1 are autoimmune in that they recognize and attack their own IgE or IgE receptor.

In the autoimmune form of hives, antibodies are made that recognize and trigger allergic cells to release histamine and other chemicals of allergy that cause hives. Some people also develop hives in response to cold temperature, contact with cold (like an ice cube), sweating, sun exposure, scratching, heat, pressure, vibration, and water.

The most common causes of autoimmune hives result from auto-antibodies recognizing and attaching to the receptor for the antibody IgE on mast cells or the allergic antibody IgE itself. The auto-antibodies cause mast cells to release histamine and allergy-causing chemicals in the *absence* of an allergic trigger (Kaplan 2009).

If there is one episode of hives, the triggering factor is obvious, or the hives last less than six weeks, your child's symptoms were probably the result of an allergy. This is usually quite clear in the case of food, which can cause hives on ingestion and/or on contact with the skin. If your child drinks milk and has hives each and every time but does not have hives when not drinking milk, it seems fairly straightforward that milk is likely the trigger for the hives. Frequently, other signs of allergy occur at the same time when this exposure occurs.

If there is no clear cause or the condition continues for more than six weeks, the cause is usually autoimmune. When it is autoimmune, any circumstance that causes the immune system to be in high gear and make more antibodies—illness, allergic reaction, times of stress, and, very rarely, arthritis or cancer—may cause the hives to flare.

Diagnosing Hives

Some tests we might perform include allergy testing, especially if you, as a parent, suspect an allergy or we suspect an allergy after we hear your medical history. Allergy is always the default pathway and the easiest problem to solve (with allergen avoidance, and/or medications, and/or allergy immunotherapy), so we check that first. As part of the initial work-up, we may also check for signs of other autoimmune diseases that tend to accompany chronic hives with basic blood counts, kidney and liver tests, tests for inflammation, and thyroid tests.

Additional tests for autoimmunity are given when the initial testing results point toward that possibility or if the trigger is unclear. Occasionally, if we are uncertain whether the rash is hives, we may request a skin biopsy. We may also request additional tests if we mutually decide to start certain medications (see below). Some patients experience an exacerbation of symptoms on ingestion of aspirin or non-steroidal anti-inflammatory drugs (like naproxen, ibuprofen, aspirin, and indomethacin) or opioid analgesics (like hydrocodone or oxycodone). It is important to avoid these drugs when possible.

Avoid ACE Inhibitors If Your Child Has Angioedema

Those patients with hives who have accompanying swelling, or angioedema, especially of the throat and tongue, should also avoid medications of the "angiotensin-converting enzyme (ACE) inhibitor" or "angiotensin receptor blocker (ARB)" classes. These are typically used for blood pressure control and sometimes for kidney protection in diabetes. While excellent medications for these issues, events such as hives, swelling, and cough are side effects that are unanticipated and should be discontinued until the problem resolves. Some patients can tolerate a similar medication or a slightly different class (9.4%) but there is risk of recurrence and there is also a risk from switching to a similar class (2-17%).

Anti-H1 Histamines

When you are having a flare and your allergic cells are releasing histamines and leukotrienes, antihistamines (like Benadryl) and anti-leukotrienes are used to mask the symptoms. Medications effective for two of the four known histamine receptors are available over-the-counter. Primary side effects of these medications are dryness of the eyes, mouth, and skin, reflux symptoms or gastrointestinal discomfort, and sedation for some (see Table 2, Anti-H1 Histamines, Chapter 8).

Precautions when taking antihistamines:

- Antihistamines should not be taken in excess. Follow your allergist-immunologist's recommendation or the instructions on the package insert if you haven't spoken to your allergist yet.
- Antihistamines should not be taken with some common antibiotics because the combination can cause a heart rhythm disturbance that, although rare, can be fatal.
- Patients with prostate problems should be cautious taking antihistamines because they can exacerbate symptoms of an enlarged prostate. This is very rare in children.
- Allergy is always a potential, albeit rare, side effect of all antihistamine H1 medications.
- Antihistamines can increase the risk of dehydration.
- Antihistamines change mood and sleep ability.
- Long-term use of antihistamines may lead to memory issues and dementia.

Anti-H2 Histamines

The second type of antihistamine medication, anti-H2, is most commonly used for indigestion. See Table 3 in Chapter 8 for a list of these over-the-counter drugs. Use according to the manufacturer's recommendations, doses, and follow their precautions.

Anti-Leukotrienes

When the mast cells recognize allergies and get stimulated, they release histamines—but they also release other chemicals. Leukotrienes are chemicals with similar effects as histamine that we can specifically block.

Anti-leukotrienes block the other big chemicals that are released from the mast cell granules during an allergic reaction. In my experience, anti-leukotriene agents are extremely effective for some patients and not helpful at all for others. It takes roughly one month of daily use to determine if they are effective. They are always used in conjunction with antihistaminergic receptor blockers as they would not likely be effective alone (see Table 4 in Chapter 8).

Limitations of anti-leukotrienes

Regrettably, anti-leukotrienes never actually solve the problem of the allergic reaction; they help control the symptoms. Even then, anti-leukotrienes are frequently insufficient for remission of autoimmune hives. Many patients need to take mild forms of chemotherapy to put them in remission from hives. Because chemotherapy involves stronger drugs designed to suppress the immune system, they have more side effects and are not for everyone.

Important recommendation – epinephrine can help during a severe episode of hives

If your physician prescribed epinephrine during an episode of hives out of concern about possible impairment of the airway, it is meant for your protection. If your throat begins to close, you feel like passing out, or you are very frightened, use your epinephrine pen immediately, call 911, and go to the emergency room as soon as possible.

Avoid Chronic Use of Steroids

Corticosteroids, like prednisone, are commonly prescribed for hives. They work very rapidly and are known to help but may not be sufficient to put your hives in remission. Using them frequently or in high doses can be problematic due to their many side effects, which include but are not limited to problems with the bones, joints, muscles, blood sugar control, blood pressure, and cholesterol control.

Your child's own adrenal glands make corticosteroids daily to help control many of his/her essential metabolic processes. However, when oral corticosteroids are used, your child's adrenal glands can stop producing them and, ultimately, stop working permanently, making them steroid-dependent or causing death. Therefore, it is best to avoid the use of systemic corticosteroids except when throat closure or airway compromise occurs.

Chapter 11

Allergic Rhinitis from Food: Please Pass the Dish (and the Tissues)

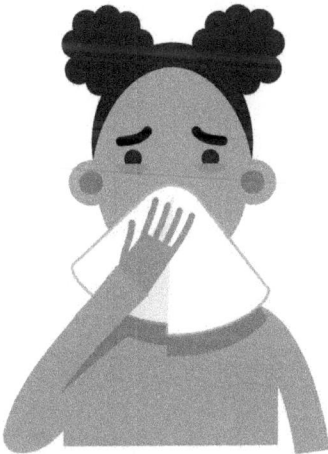

I've had many patients who have the embarrassing symptom of a runny nose after they eat. Several patients identified specific foods that they thought were causative and, after validating their suspicions by avoiding those foods in potentially embarrassing situations, they found great relief. Because a runny nose is not life-threatening, I do not endorse complete avoidance of the suspected food because an intolerance may develop.

Allergic rhinitis is a group of symptoms generally attributed to pollen. These familiar symptoms from hay fever include nasal congestion, postnasal drip, rhinorrhea, itchy, red, and runny eyes, coughing, and sneezing. In fact, allergic rhinitis from food is thought to be secondary to pollen and the result of cross-reactivity. In other words, similarity of a pollen protein to a food protein results in allergic reaction to both. Allergic rhinitis to food is thought to be due to the same cross-reactivities that cause oral allergy syndrome (see Chapter 12).

Symptoms of Allergic Rhinitis

Allergenic foods can cause a drippy nose and can lead to post-nasal drip and cough as well as eye symptoms of redness, itchiness, and lacrimation. This tends to be one of a number of different symptoms. Rice, citrus fruits, and bananas are some of the most commonly implicated foods.

There is also a form of nonallergic rhinitis, known as gustatory rhinitis, that can be triggered by foods such as milk, dairy products, and wine. Acid reflux after eating can also cause rhinitis, postnasal drip, and coughing.

Testing of Allergic Rhinitis

Blood tests and/or skin tests can be performed to diagnose allergic rhinitis.

Treatment of Allergic Rhinitis

Treatment involves avoidance of the food to reduce or eliminate uncomfortable symptoms.

Chapter 12

Oral Allergy Syndrome:
A Mouthful of Allergies

Oral allergy syndrome (OAS) is a mild form of allergy that occurs upon contact of the mouth and throat with raw fruits or vegetables, causing itching and swelling of the mouth, face, lips, tongue, and throat (AAAAI 2020). When a person with a pollen allergy reacts to certain foods and/or substances—called cross-reactivity—the OAS is called pollen fruit syndrome (PFS).

Symptoms of OAS

The itching, tingling, or swelling reaction is usually limited to the oral cavity and tends to happen while the food is still in the mouth and oral cavity. Symptoms may be specific to a particular variety of fruit or vegetable and/or to a particular stage of ripeness. In rare cases, OAS can lead to anaphylaxis.

Heating Trigger Foods Can Reduce Cross-Reactions

Besides avoiding your trigger food(s), baking food may decrease the risk of allergic reaction, because high temperatures break down the proteins responsible for OAS. Eating canned food may also limit the reaction. Peeling the food before eating may also be helpful, as the offending protein is often concentrated in the skin.

Testing for OAS

Testing may not be necessary if you know your child's specific trigger foods and avoid them. However, if unexpected reactions are occurring, it may be necessary to test.

Skin and/or blood testing is done for specific pollen and foods. We may test both fresh and processed foods because the processed food may yield a negative reaction whereas a prick-prick test with fresh fruits or vegetables will likely be positive.

Treatment for OAS

Seek help if your child's symptoms become anaphylactic or life-threatening. If cooking ameliorates the symptoms, always be sure to thoroughly cook the trigger food(s) or eat the trigger food only if it has been processed by baking or canning.

You should talk to your allergist-immunologist if your child's OAS symptoms are:

- causing significant throat discomfort, like they are choking or cannot swallow;
- are getting worse;
- are caused by cooked fruits and vegetables or nuts, as these have a greater risk of becoming life-threatening; and/or
- your child shows signs of anaphylaxis like hives, vomiting, or difficulty breathing, after eating raw fruits and vegetables.

◆ ◆ ◆

Before I was an allergist-immunologist, I noticed that every August, my mouth would itch when I ate honeydew melon, especially when it was just becoming ripe. And when I say itchy, I mean I would have agreed to rub my tongue against tree bark—it was that severe. My inner ears, just beyond reach of a cotton swab, were also unbelievably itchy. Cantaloupe also made me itch, but less so. The itch was so severe I would have described it as painful. Before and after August, there was no issue. This is because ragweed—which has strong cross-reactivity with melons—pollinates in August. By the way, I never had issues with watermelon, banana, cucumbers, white potatoes, or zucchini, but that is how cross-reactivity works (see fig. 33 below). It is possible to react to multiple foods but it's not likely that you'd react to all foods in a cross-reactive group.

Interestingly, this only happened for a few years and has not occurred since. But I am still very cautious to avoid ripe honeydew melon during an intense and/or peak ragweed season. I just have to look at honeydew melons and I am overcome with nausea. Once you finish reading this book, you will recognize my response as a food aversion from a previous negative experience because it does not cause problems for me anymore.

◆ ◆ ◆

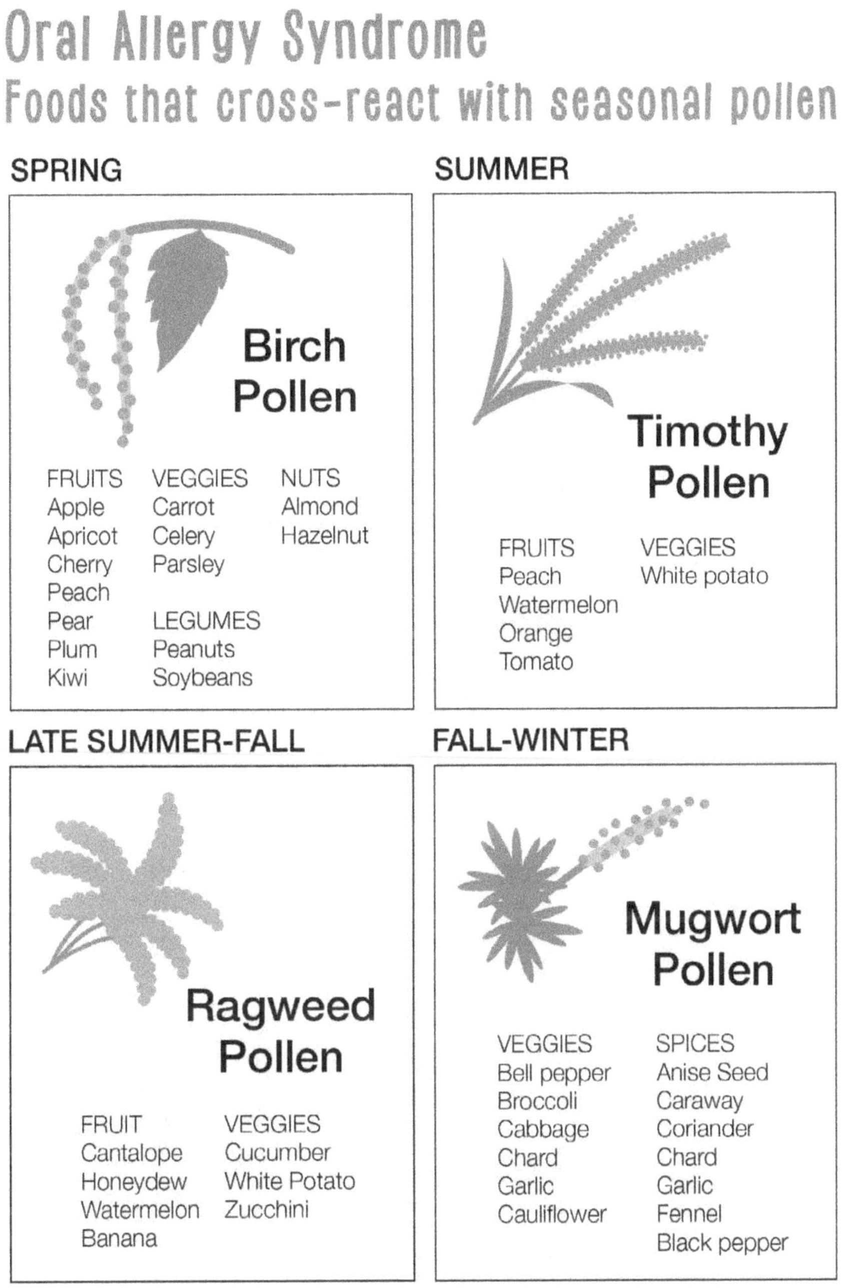

Oral Allergy Syndrome
Foods that cross-react with seasonal pollen

SPRING

Birch Pollen

FRUITS	VEGGIES	NUTS
Apple	Carrot	Almond
Apricot	Celery	Hazelnut
Cherry	Parsley	
Peach		
Pear	LEGUMES	
Plum	Peanuts	
Kiwi	Soybeans	

SUMMER

Timothy Pollen

FRUITS	VEGGIES
Peach	White potato
Watermelon	
Orange	
Tomato	

LATE SUMMER-FALL

Ragweed Pollen

FRUIT	VEGGIES
Cantalope	Cucumber
Honeydew	White Potato
Watermelon	Zucchini
Banana	

FALL-WINTER

Mugwort Pollen

VEGGIES	SPICES
Bell pepper	Anise Seed
Broccoli	Caraway
Cabbage	Coriander
Chard	Chard
Garlic	Garlic
Cauliflower	Fennel
	Black pepper

Figure 35: Patterns of Oral Allergy Syndrome: The specific foods that demonstrate cross reactivity with pollen allergens of the spring, summer, late summer-fall, and fall-winter.

Chapter 13

Alpha-Gal Allergy:
A Contagious Allergy

Alpha-gal allergy is a severe and potentially life-threatening allergy to a carbohydrate molecule (galactose-alpha-1,3-galactose) found in most mammalian or red meat. Unlike other food allergy reactions that typically occur within minutes of ingestion, symptoms from eating red meat such as pork, lamb, or beef may be delayed, occurring three to eight hours after eating.

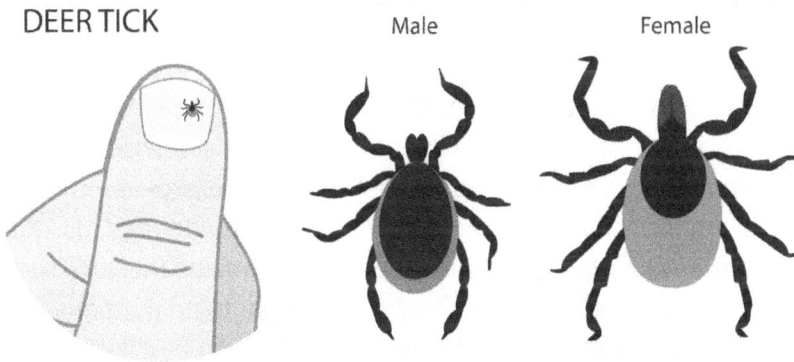

DEER TICK   Male   Female

Figure 36: This tiny insect may carry a contagious allergy to red meat.

Alpha-gal is unique as an allergen for several reasons. First, this allergy is transmitted by the Lone Star tick that exposes the patient to the alpha-galactose present in their saliva when it feeds on humans. This exposure sensitizes people and results in an anaphylactic response to one or more mammalian meats when consumed. This is because typical mammalian meats—beef, pork, venison, rabbit, lamb, or other mammalian products—may contain alpha-gal sugar. In contrast, alpha-gal is not found in fish, reptiles, birds, or people. In contrast to most food allergies, the time of onset of anaphylaxis from alpha-gal may be variable and is delayed if the meat is consumed with fat.

Symptoms of Alpha-Gal

- The allergic reaction occurs during the digestive process—three to eight hours after eating—with increasing time directly proportional to the increased amount of fat in the meal. Common symptoms are:
- hives and itching
- swelling of your child's lips, face, or eyelids
- shortness of breath, cough, or wheezing
- abdominal pain, nausea, diarrhea, or vomiting

The most severe reaction, anaphylaxis, can present as a combination of several of these symptoms, may include low blood pressure, and is potentially fatal (AAAAI 2019).

Testing for Alpha-Gal

Your child's allergist may recommend testing that includes skin tests to the relevant animal proteins and blood tests which measure the levels of a specific immunoglobulin E (IgE) antibody to galactose-alpha-1,3-galactose and to the specific mammalian meats in a patient's diet.

Treatment for Alpha-Gal

Immediate symptoms such as hives or shortness of breath are treated the same as any other food allergy, in an urgent care setting with antihistamines, epinephrine, and other medications. It is now appreciated that alpha-gal allergy does not always include every mammalian meat. Therefore, testing for allergy to the individual meats is necessary to prevent a restricted diet. Avoidance of the meats that provoke an allergic reaction is necessary. This allergy was originally thought to be permanent but as time has progressed since its discovery, it is known that it can be "outgrown" or lessen over time for some patients. Until this occurs, patients that suffer with this are best advised to take all anaphylaxis precautions.

Unfortunately, this allergy is not known to be responsive to food oral immunotherapy (FOIT).

I've diagnosed several patients with this and it is always an interesting surprise, as the event of being bitten with a tick is never connected with meat allergy. It really is one of our most bizarre allergies.

Prevention of Alpha-Gal

The only long-term solution is to avoid the trigger: mammalian meat. Your child can still enjoy chicken and fish because they don't cause similar reactions.

I do recommend regular testing for alpha-gal, as I have noticed over the years that this condition can change and the range of allergic meats can narrow. However, as it may take years to resolve and may not resolve at all (we still do not know enough to answer with certainty), I recommend re-testing every year or every other year.

You may be advised to carry an epinephrine auto-injector for your child, to be used in case of subsequent accidental exposures and reaction.

Part 3: Non-IgE Mediated Allergy

Stop Hating Your Guts: Delayed Hypersensitivity Reactions Injure The Intestinal Tract

Chapter Preview

- Which food allergies are linked to intestinal tract injury and inflammation?
- How are delayed hypersensitivity reactions diagnosed?
- This type of allergic reaction includes celiac disease, dermatitis herpetiformis, and systemic contact dermatitis.
- How are these allergies managed?

Heating Trigger Foods Can Reduce Cross-Reactions

Non-IgE mediated immune system injury, also known as delayed hypersensitivity reactions, generally implicates cells that attack various parts of the intestine and cause injury. Because the cells take longer to activate and migrate to the area where they cause damage, these allergies are called Type IV or delayed hypersensitivity reactions.

Most non-IgE mediated allergy syndromes are diagnosed by patient history, as no simple, valid tests are widely available for these disorders. Empirically eliminating the consumption of the suspected food with resulting elimination of the symptoms is the most typical and efficient method used to test and treat simultaneously. In some cases, patch testing may be used to identify the triggering food.

Patch testing involves placing chambers containing the suspected foods in contact with the skin. Forty-eight hours after placement, the allergist-immunologist removes the patches and examines any sign of skin irritation or allergy to the substances. A second reading occurs about one week after placement, when the allergist-immunologist assesses the allergy's severity by measuring the extent of the rash (see Chapter 17 for details about ROAT testing for sensitive skin).

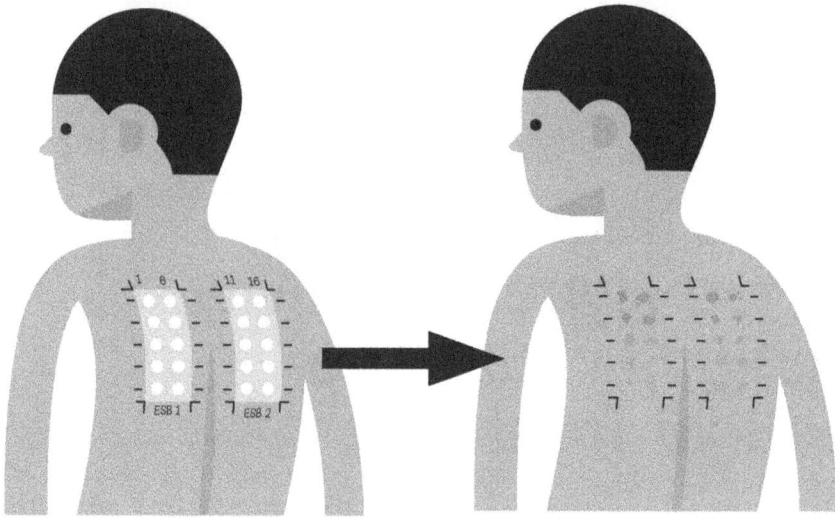

Figure 37: Patch testing is sometimes used to test for food sensitivities. Patches of potential allergens are placed on the back of the patient and then removed after approximately 48 hours. The reaction of the skin is noted and recorded during this "first read." Approximately seven days after the patches are placed, a "second read" is conducted and the skin reaction is noted a second time.

Treatment Involves Identification of the Trigger and Avoidance

Ultimately, avoidance of the triggering substance is necessary for the long-term comfort and safety of the patient who has a non-IgE mediated food allergy.

While those allergic triggers are being identified, treatment may include topical or oral steroids to control the inflammation and may include antihistamines to control itching in cases of dermatitis. In cases of gastrointestinal issues, avoidance is the cornerstone of treatment and topical steroids are used for some syndromes.

When patients with eczema or delayed food allergy are not completely satisfied with their progress despite avoiding their food allergies and aggressively addressing their environmental allergies, I recommend patch testing to see if a delayed allergy may be a trigger. This is an alternative to removing the allergen from the diet to determine if symptoms evolve. Effectively, they both test the delayed allergy, but one technique might be preferred to another in terms of comfort or efficiency.

Chapter 15

Celiac Disease: Gut Feeling

Chapter Preview

- The many different health conditions that may accompany celiac disease.
- What is the gold standard test for diagnosing celiac disease?
- What are the most effective treatment methods?

Celiac disease (CD) is a non-IgE-mediated gluten allergy or hypersensitivity. This food-protein-induced small intestinal disease goes by multiple names, including gluten enteropathy, celiac sprue, sprue, and celiac disease. Symptoms may include chronic diarrhea and signs of malabsorption in the part of the gut that absorbs iron, frequently resulting in iron-deficiency anemia.

Health Implications of Celiac Disease

The malabsorptive process, in addition to causing iron deficiency, can also cause deficiencies of B12, calcium, vitamin K, vitamin D, zinc, and copper. Symptomatically, these deficiencies can result in mouth sores; fatigue and irritability; numbness and tingling, as well as other neurologic issues due to malabsorption of B12; inability to gain weight as well as weight loss; delayed growth in children; thin bones contributing to osteoporosis, fractures, and discolored teeth; lactose intolerance, bloating, and gas; headaches and even migraines; depression; and anxiety. Malaise and fatigue are common as a secondary result of many of these issues.

- The most common abnormality of celiac disease is mild to moderate elevation of liver function tests, known as the transaminases, which indicates liver damage. This damage can be present without other symptoms of liver disease.
- Low albumin and prolonged coagulation times from low vitamin K levels may result from malabsorption and intestinal inflammation.
- The enteropathy (inflammation of the intestine) results in leakage through the gut wall, causing loss of protein in general. Unfortunately, that includes loss of globulins (immunoglobulin or antibodies) which flag foreign bacterial invaders

to prevent infection. As a result, recurrent infections of the respiratory system and of the ear can occur.

- Other symptoms include joint pain, liver disease, dermatitis herpetiformis (celiac skin rash; see Chapter 16), and infertility by adulthood.
- Dermatitis herpetiformis (DH) is the classic rash of celiac disease, which appears as highly itchy clusters of vesicles and typically involves the extensor surfaces of the lower extremities more than the upper extremities. DH may be the only physical sign of the disease.

Celiac disease is present in 3 million Americans, or 1 in 133 people (Beyond Celiac). In most patients, it is undiagnosed or the diagnosis is delayed.

Effect of celiac disease on intestinal lining

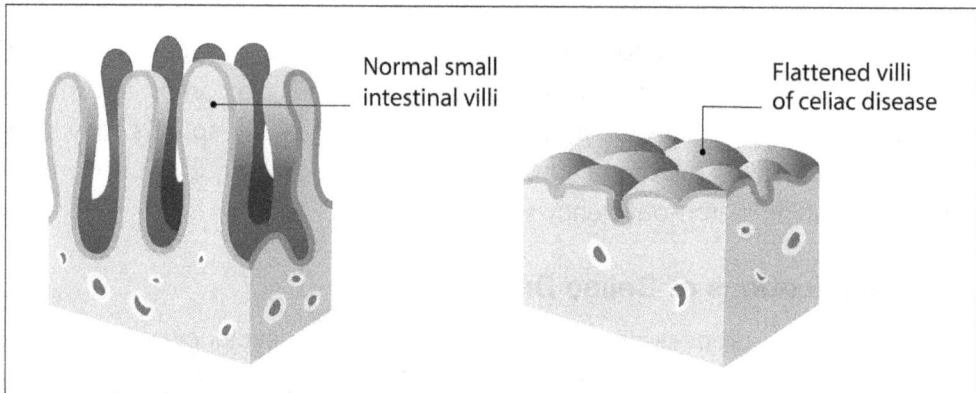

Figure 38: The damage that occurs in celiac disease results in flattening of the intestinal villi that are important for nutritional absorption.

Diagnosis of Celiac Disease

Diagnosis can be made by assessing levels of autoimmune antibodies or by biopsy of the small intestine, demonstrating villous flattening. Intestinal biopsy is the gold standard for diagnosis of CD. The serum tests detect increased levels of anti-gliadin and anti-tissue transglutaminase antibody levels. These levels are less reliable in the presence of background liver disease and low or absent IgA in the immune system, which can lead to false positive or false negative results, respectively. These proteins, which are present in wheat, also cross react with the small intestine, resulting in damage. This makes celiac disease an autoimmune disease, a disease in which the immune system turns against the patient's body and attacks specific areas, resulting in damage. In this case the cross-reactive proteins (and the damage) are in the small intestine.

Treatment involves a strict and permanent fast from gluten, which is present in wheat, rye, oat, barley, and many other products that use wheat as an ingredient or in processing. If test results are negative, consider exploring alternatives to what might be occurring with your child's allergist-immunologist. Even if your child doesn't have celiac disease, it does not mean he/she is not suffering.

Complications Common to Celiac Disease

Some patients with celiac disease also have health risks not clearly linked to their gluten sensitivity. These complications include an elevated risk of intestinal lymphoma and small bowel cancer. Other complications, including neurological issues such as peripheral neuropathy, malnutrition, osteoporosis, and defects in tooth enamel are related to malnutrition, intestinal inflammation, and increased gut permeability.

Patients' CD refractory to a gluten-free diet can have lactose intolerance (as well as difficulty digesting other sugars), pancreatic insufficiency, irritable bowel syndrome, microscopic colitis, and bacterial overgrowth. In children, short stature and delayed puberty may be the presenting symptoms.

Uncontrolled celiac may provoke other autoimmune processes, which may be triggered by the antibody flags cross-reacting with other tissue. When this occurs and causes damage, it may result in thyroid disease, diabetes, or other autoimmune diseases.

Several cancers are associated with celiac disease: a type of T-cell lymphoma, non-Hodgkin's lymphoma, and small intestinal adenocarcinoma (Rubio-Tapia, 2013). It is thought that the chronic inflammation eventually leads to these rare cancers in these patients.

Testing for Celiac Disease

There are several ways to diagnose celiac disease, including blood testing and biopsy of the small intestine (see Table 9). Two to three percent of patients with celiac have negative blood tests (CDC; NIDDK 2021).

For patients with IgA deficiency and those with negative celiac disease blood test results with highly suspicious symptoms, it is wise to have an upper endoscopy with biopsies of the duodenal bulb to attempt diagnosis of celiac disease. This is because one of the important auto-antibodies that aids in diagnosis is an IgA antibody. In IgA deficiency, very few to none of these autoantibodies are made, making this blood test unreliable.

Table 9

Diagnostic Tests for Celiac Disease	
Tissue transglutaminase tTG-IgA and IgA tests	This is an inaccurate test for patients with IgA deficiency and for patients under two, due to lower levels of IgA at that age (Rubio-Tapia, 2013). Both tests must be done at the same time. 4% false positive rate, 7% false negative rate.
IgA endomysial antibody (EMA)	Test has 0% false positive rate, 5-10% false negative rate.
Deamidated gliadin peptide antibodies	This is a preferred test if the tTG results are thought to be falsely negative or if the patient has IgA deficiency. Anti-DGP IgA sensitivity of 92.4% and specificity of 97.6% and an Anti-DGP IgG sensitivity of 97.8 and specificity of 97.6%.
Upper endoscopy with biopsy of small intestine	Under previous guidelines and without duodenal bulb biopsy. False negative rate may be as high as 9-13%.
Video capsule endoscopy	Better than endoscopy at detecting macroscopic atrophy and complications. Test has 5% false positive rate, 11% false negative rate.
Intestinal fatty acid binding protein (I-FABP)	I-FABP is present inside cells and when found in the blood, can be an indicator of cell injury from gluten intake. Test not widely available.
Genetic testing (HLA-DQ2 and HLA-DQ8)	Tests must be performed together to achieve the 99% negative predictive value of this test. 25-30% of U.S. population tests positive for either one or the other. Test has 0% false positive rate, 20% false negative rate.
Radiology	Radiology may suggest findings that have been associated with celiac disease, such as small bowel dilatation, wall thickening, vascular changes. These findings are not necessarily diagnostic in themselves but may prompt further evaluation.

Adapted from following resources:
Laposata M, Nichols JH, Steele P, Stricker TP, Sarkar MK. Methods. In: Laposata M. eds. *Laposata's Laboratory Medicine: Diagnosis of Disease in the Clinical Laboratory*, 3rd ed. McGraw Hill; 2019. Accessed December 13, 2022. https://accessmedicine.mhmedical.com/content.aspx?bookid=2503&sectionid=201361411
Ratner, Amy. At-home test for celiac disease launches. Beyond Celiac website. Updated December 5, 2018. Accessed December 12, 2022. https://www.beyondceliac.org/research-news/at-home-test-for-celiac-disease-launches/

In this situation, endoscopy is more reliable because immune system damage results in flattening of the normally finger-like villi, which is the expected finding on biopsy. This may not be apparent if the patient has fasted from gluten during the biopsy, as fasting normalizes the small intestine; the autoantibodies stop attacking with no exposure to wheat or other gluten. Once diagnosed, endoscopy and biopsy are used to track effectiveness of diet and screen for the cancers that, while rare, are more likely in patients with celiac disease.

Genetic testing to HLA-DQ2.5 and HLA-DQ8, one or the other of which is present in celiac disease, can be used to rule out celiac disease or screen relatives for their potential to develop celiac disease. 95% of patients with celiac have HLA-DQ 2.5 and 5% have HLA-DQ8 (Rubio-Tapia 2013). However, it is believed that in addition to the presence of one or both of these genes, a second insult is required to cause celiac. The nature of this insult is unknown but may be something like a viral exposure or extreme stress of some kind.

Treatment for Celiac

Celiac disease is not outgrown. Treatment requires lifetime avoidance of gluten in wheat, rye, and barley. Sometimes other grains such as oats are incriminated, but only because they may be contaminated by the gluten-containing grains they contact in processing. In people who haven't had any celiac symptoms for at least six months, eating moderate amounts of pure, non-contaminated oats seems to be safe (Medline Plus 2021a). Safe grains include brown, black, or wild rice, quinoa, amaranth, pure buckwheat, corn, cornmeal, popcorn, millet, gluten-free oats, sorghum, and teff (Medline Plus 2021b).

Monitoring

It is recommended that celiac patients have the following monitored by their healthcare provider:

- Celiac disease antibodies (tTG - IgA (see Table 9)
- Nutritional anemia profile (hemoglobin, hematocrit, folate, ferritin, vitamin B12)
- Vitamin profile (thiamine, vitamin B6, 25-hydroxy vitamin D)
- Mineral profile (copper, zinc)
- Lipid profile
- Electrolyte and renal profile
- Complete blood count (CBC)
- Thyroid stimulating hormone (TSH)
- DEXA bone scan for osteopenia/osteoporosis

Chapter 16

Dermatitis Herpetiformis: Getting Rid of Your Wheat Rash

Dermatitis herpetiformis is a skin rash consisting of intensely itchy clusters of blisters and is the skin manifestation of celiac disease. It is triggered by Immunoglobulin A—the autoantibody of celiac disease in the skin and the one typically found in mucosal membranes—being deposited into the dermal layer (the layer under the epidermis).

Average age at diagnosis is 30-40 years old. While it can occur anytime, it is more common in males and rare in young children. It can be diagnosed via biopsy. Treatment is avoidance of gluten. Some patients require dapsone medication to help put this skin rash in remission.

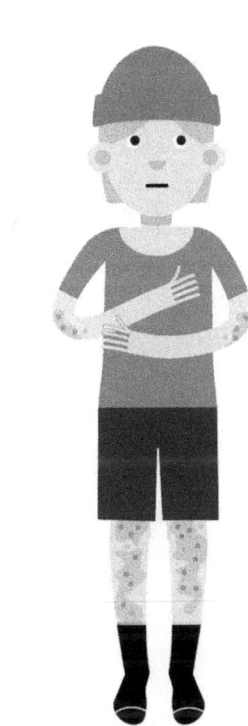

Figure 39: Dermatitis herpetiformis predominantly affects elbows, knees, buttocks, and scalp.

Chapter 17

Systemic Contact Dermatitis: Last Week's Dinner, This Week's Rash

Chapter Preview

- What are the common allergens and foods that cause contact dermatitis?
- What is the difference between contact dermatitis and systemic contact dermatitis? What causes it to become systemic?
- What are the symptoms of systemic contact dermatitis and how are they treated?

Examples of Contact Dermatitis Triggers

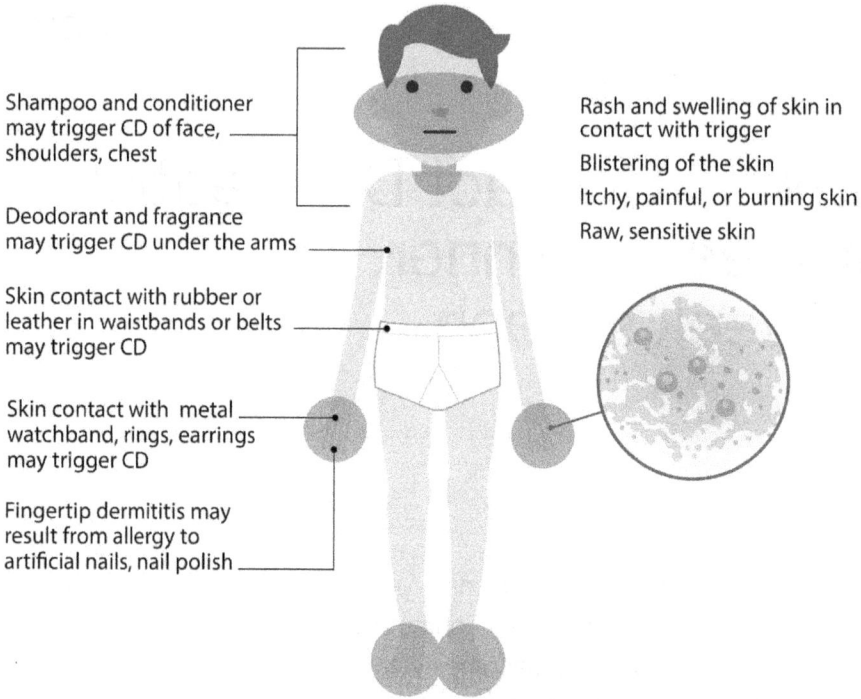

Shampoo and conditioner may trigger CD of face, shoulders, chest

Deodorant and fragrance may trigger CD under the arms

Skin contact with rubber or leather in waistbands or belts may trigger CD

Skin contact with metal watchband, rings, earrings may trigger CD

Fingertip dermititis may result from allergy to artificial nails, nail polish

Rash and swelling of skin in contact with trigger

Blistering of the skin

Itchy, painful, or burning skin

Raw, sensitive skin

Figure 40: Examples of contact dermatitis triggers.

Systemic contact dermatitis is one of many delayed response types of allergies. Contact dermatitis is an itchy rash located where the skin comes into contact with the allergen. It can also present as a red, itchy, or burning rash around the mouth (perioral) or rectum (perirectal), as well as stomach irritation.

The most common culprits are the most common food allergies overall, which include peanuts, tree nuts, wheat, eggs, soy, fish, shellfish, and sesame. Other allergic triggers include plant and herbal products, preservatives, excipients, cosmetics, medications, and metals.

How a Contact Allergy Becomes Systemic

A contact allergy can become systemic when a person who is already exposed and sensitized to an allergen is exposed to the allergen via a systemic route, such as ingestion, inhalation, sublingual, or intravenous or intramuscular injection.

Symptoms of systemic contact dermatitis can present as a flare of the rash at the original rash or testing site and may spread over large areas of the body. Other systemic side effects that may occur include nausea, vomiting, diarrhea, fatigue, headache, and fever.

There are several characteristic rashes of systemic contact dermatitis. Baboon syndrome is when erythema and rash present on the buttocks, much like the red buttocks of a baboon. It is believed the cause is a new reaction to a systemic exposure, most commonly a drug, that has previously had contact with the skin.

Another presentation of systemic contact dermatitis is a vesicular dermatitis that is a form of dyshidrotic eczema. Most commonly affected parts of the body are the hands and the feet.

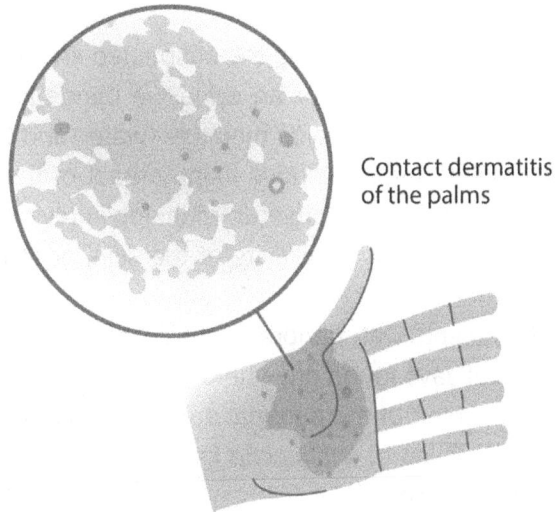

Contact dermatitis of the palms

Figure 41: Contact dermatitis of the palms.

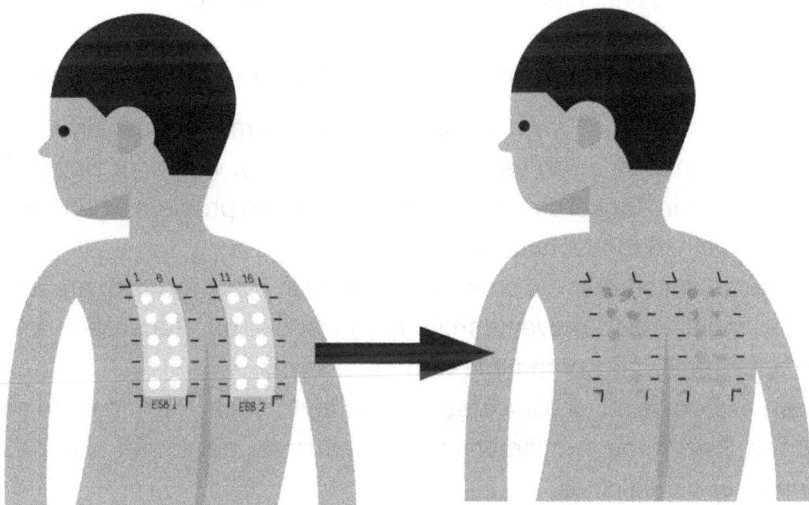

Figure 42: Patch testing involves placing suspected substances in contact with the skin—usually on the back—to discover which substances trigger a skin reaction.

Testing for Systemic Contact Dermatitis

The primary testing method for systemic contact dermatitis is patch testing, which involves placing chambers containing suspected drugs, foods, chemicals, or other substances in contact with the skin.

For my patients with "sensitive skin," I usually recommend ROAT testing (Repeat Open Application Test) of any new topical products prior to beginning home use. A ROAT is similar to the patch test in that the suspected substance is placed in contact with the skin for a period of time.

ROAT testing is performed by applying the suspected substance to the skin and covering it with hypoallergenic gauze or an adhesive bandage once per day for a week. During that week, the patient avoids moisture, water, and sweating in the testing area so as not to disrupt the continuous skin contact of the potential trigger or triggers. At the end of the week, the allergist-immunologist reviews the condition and extent of the rash to determine the sensitivity of the skin, enabling them to provide medical guidance.

I have had multiple patients with perioral rashes that were caused by contact allergy to food. The rash is always found anywhere the child places the food in contact with the skin. Rashes or itching of the perianal area can many times be attributed to this allergy. It is always gratifying to see a child free of these painful rashes with elimination of one food from their diet.

Treatment of Systemic Contact Dermatitis

Treatment begins with identification of the allergic trigger(s) and subsequent avoidance of those foods or substances. In the interim, topical steroids are used to control the inflammation and antihistamines used to control itching.

Other Common Allergens in Foods That Cause Contact Dermatitis

Nickel is the most common metal to cause contact dermatitis, usually in the form of a rash where an item such as an earring, piece of jewelry, watch, or zipper has been in contact with the skin. Nickel can also create a systemic problem when it is consumed in the form of canned foods, nuts, etc.

Sorbic acid (or sorbate) is a preservative used in many foods to prevent growth of bacteria and mold; it also prevents fruits from discoloring. Because it does not have color, taste, or smell, it is compatible with most foods.

Balsam of Peru is an oil harvested in Central America. Many people are exposed to Balsam of Peru through cosmetics and perfumes, but it can also be present in foods, drinks, and medicines.

Propylene glycol was made famous by the Pfizer COVID-19 vaccine. It is also present as an excipient in other vaccines and medicines where it is used to stabilize

the components. It is also present in some antihistamine tablets, so if your child feels worse after taking one, it could be the propylene glycol.

Sensitization to **ethylenediamine**, a preservative found in many creams and cosmetics, may also lead to cross-sensitivity to ethylene-diamine-tetra-acetic acid (EDTA), a preservative in many foods.

Reactivity to the plants and pollen of the **compositae** plant family—arnica, German chamomile, and herbal remedies—may create skin or systemic reactions upon exposure to many of the plant family's vegetables and herbs.

Parabens are a common preservative, widely used in cosmetics, pharmaceuticals, and foods.

Formaldehyde is used for its preservation and bleaching traits in cosmetics, paints, and textiles. It is also naturally occurring in many foods. Aspartame sweetener is metabolized into formaldehyde by the body. Because it is water soluble, it is easy to wash off with water. Formalin, used in many countries as a preservative, can be metabolized to formaldehyde.

Table 10

Common Food Ingredients That Cause Contact Dermatitis				
Food	Balsam of Peru	Chromium	Cobalt	Compositae
Apricots			x	
Artichoke				x
Bananas, grapes, apples				
Beans, legumes			x	
Beer			x	
Beets			x	
Breads		x	x	
Brewer's yeast		x		
Broccoli		x	x	
Cake mixes		x	x	
Canned produce				x (some)
Carrots				
Cereals			x	
Cheeses				
Chocolate	x		x	
Cinnamon	x			
Citrus	x			
Cloves	x		x	
Cocoa			x	
Coffee, tea			x	
Colas	x			
Dairy				
Dressings				x (some)
Dried fruit				x (some)
Dried mushroom				
Dried soups				
Endive				x
Fish, scallops			x	
Food coloring				
Frozen dairy	x			
Fruit preservatives with sorbate				x (some)
Grape juice		x		
Green beans		x		

EDTA	Formaldehyde	Nickel	Parabens	Polyethylene glycol	Sorbate
	x				
		x			
x	x		x		x
				x	
				x	
x					x
	x				
					x
		x			
		x (limited)*			
		x			
		x			
				x	
				x	
				x	
					x
	x				
				x	
			x		
	x	x (some)			x
				x	
			x		
					x

Table 11

Common Food Ingredients That Cause Contact Dermatitis				
Food	Balsam of Peru	Chromium	Cobalt	Compositae
Green, leafy vegetables			x	
Jams				x
Lettuce			x	x
Margarine				
Meat		x		
Medicines	x (some)			
Mussels		x		
Nuts			x	
Oats, oatmeal			x	
Onions, garlic				
Packaged, frozen foods				x (some)
Pickles				
Plums				
Popcorn				
Potatoes		x		
Red wine		x		
Syrups				
Teas***				x
Tuna, herring, salmon, mackerel, shellfish				
Utensils with nickel				
Vanilla	x			
White wine				
Whole grain flour		x	x	
Yarrow, mugwort, echinacea				x

*Especially when used with nickel cooking utensils.
**Especially when used with acidic foods.
***Specifically, chamomile, chrysanthemum, sunflower.

EDTA	Formaldehyde	Nickel	Parabens	Polyethylene glycol	Sorbate
	x (some)	x			
					x
		x			
					x
	x				x
	x				x
		x			
		x			
	x	x			
x				x	
			x		
	x	x			
				x	
					x
			x		
	x	x			x
		x**			
					x

Katta R, Schlichte M. Diet and dermatitis: food triggers. *J Clin Aesthet Dermatol*. 2014; 7(3):30-6. Accessed November 1, 2022. https://www.ncbi.nlm.nih.gov/pmc/articles/PMC3970830/

Part 4: Mixed Allergy

Chapter 18

Gut Reaction: Childhood Gastrointestinal System Inflammation

Chapter Preview

- Which disease states combine an immediate, intense allergic reaction and a delayed response?
- Understand which parts of the gastrointestinal system are inflamed in each disease state.
- Common food triggers.
- Management strategies to increase comfort and reduce inflammation.

Focus on the Gastrointestinal Tract

To refresh your memory, IgE-mediated food allergy is initiated by the allergic flags of the immune system known as food-specific IgE. When the trigger food latches onto the food-specific IgE and they are cross-linked, allergic cells become excited and cause chemicals to be released from the allergic cells. Those chemicals either directly damage or summon cells that create the damage. Anaphylaxis is a prime example.

Cell-mediated allergy, also known as Type IV hypersensitivity, is initiated by food-specific T cell responses. The prototypical example of cell-mediated allergy is celiac disease.

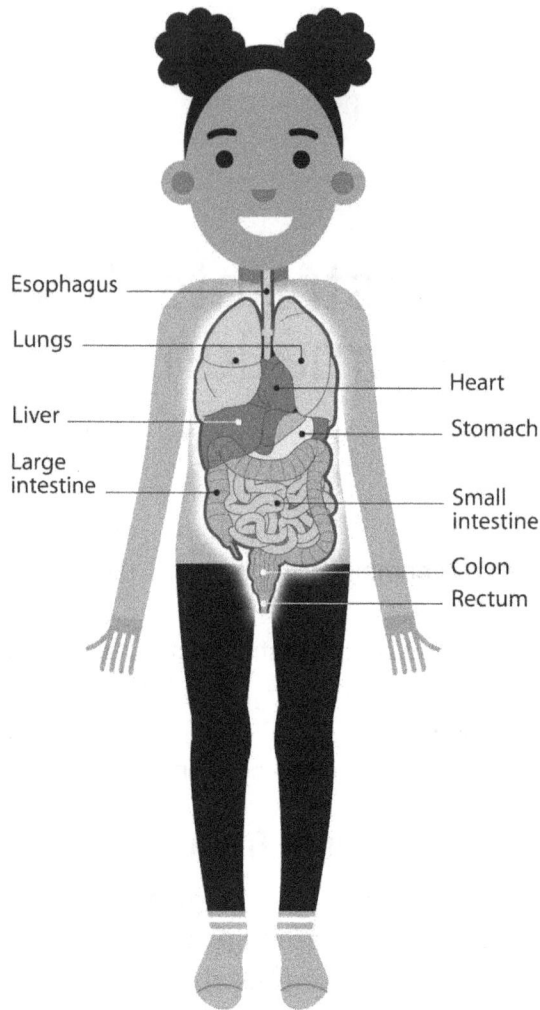

Figure 43: Normal patient anatomy. Highlighted are the parts of the gastrointestinal tract involved with mixed food allergy reaction. Closeups of each area follow.

Food Protein-Induced Enterocolitis Syndrome

Food Protein-Induced Enterocolitis Syndrome (FPIES) typically presents within the first year of life, triggered most commonly by cow's milk and soy. The prevalence in U.S. infants was 0.5% (Nowak 2019). FPIES presents as significant, often projectile and repetitive vomiting, diarrhea, dehydration, lethargy, and failure to thrive (which refers to maturation that is below normal, typically assessed by weight, height, and head circumference and suggests a problem in growth and development). It can also cause metabolic derangements, hypotension, and hypothermia.

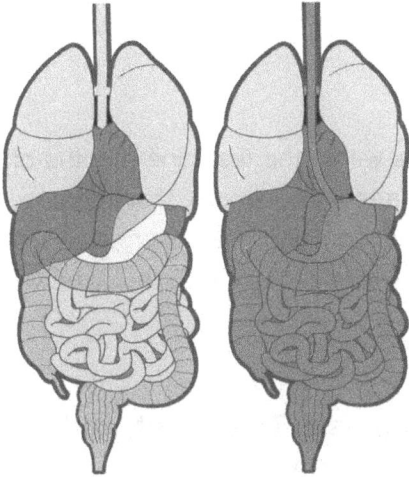

Figure 44: Left, normal digestive system. Right, inflamed gastrointestinal walls of FPIES.

Cow's milk and soy FPIES is usually diagnosed earlier and FPIES triggered by other foods starts later when these foods are typically fed to infants. There is usually only one food allergy that triggers FPIES, but, infrequently, multiple food triggers can exist.

Aside from cow's milk and soy, the most common FPIES triggers in the United States are rice, oat, wheat, corn, eggs, fish/shellfish, poultry, other meats, sweet potato, potato, squash, carrot, banana, avocado, apple, and pear.

FPIES diagnosis is challenging and might go undetected because of later onset of symptoms after food ingestion (one to four hours), lack of typical allergic skin and respiratory symptoms, and food triggers that are perceived to be hypoallergenic.

Food Protein-Induced Allergic Proctocolitis (AP)

Allergic Proctocolitis (AP) typically begins in infancy, most commonly triggered by milk and soy. As the name suggests, AP typically presents as blood-streaked, highly

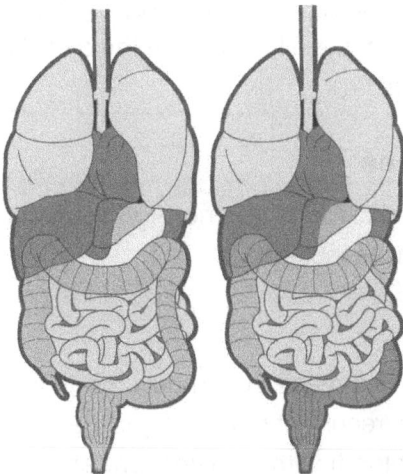

mucous stools, as well as increased gas and abdominal pain, especially on defecation. Exam shows erosions and inflammation of the rectum and anus and biopsy shows eosinophilic infiltration of these areas.

Infants with AP are typically much healthier than those with FPIES, but do have blood-streaked stool. Aside from cow's milk and soy, corn and eggs are the most implicated allergens. The prevalence of food protein-induced allergic

Figure 45: Left, normal digestive system. Right, inflamed bowel of AP.

proctocolitis is 0.16% in healthy children and 64% of patients with bloody stool (Mennini 2020).

Food Protein-Induced Enteropathy

Food Protein-Induced Enteropathy (FPE) begins within the first nine months of life, usually starting when soy or cow's milk formula is introduced. Other triggers may present later. FPE presents as refractory diarrhea, vomiting, malabsorption, and abdominal distention, as well as failure to thrive. Prevalence of FPE is unknown and thought to be decreasing (Feuille 2015).

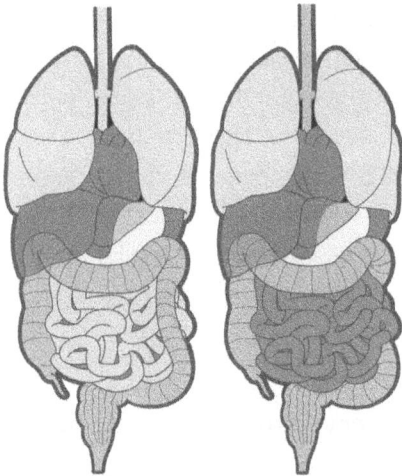

Figure 46: Left, normal digestive system. Right, inflamed small intestine of FPE.

Diagnosis, Treatment, and Resolution

Diagnosis and treatment of FPIES, AP, and FPE involves identifying and eliminating the triggering food from the diet. After a period of prolonged stability, the food is challenged to assess for resolution, which usually occurs within a few years, at which time these syndromes are typically outgrown.

Rates of FPIES remission by age six ranges from 50-90%, but the patient may be at risk for developing food allergy, possibly related to the prolonged elimination of the allergen from the diet. AP and FPE usually resolve by one to three years of age.

Childhood Reactions and Mixed Allergies

There are also non-IgE or mixed allergies to specific foods (see non-IgE mediated and mixed reaction sections, Chapter 18). Briefly, these include:

Heiner's Syndrome

Heiner's Syndrome (pulmonary hemosiderosis) is a reaction primarily triggered in infancy by cow's milk. Symptoms include chronic, recurrent respiratory issues, anemia, recurrent fever, and hemoptysis (coughing up blood) with resulting wheezing, shortness of breath, and visible pulmonary infiltrates on chest X-ray. Some children experience failure to gain weight and failure to thrive.

Presentation occurs between the ages of six months and two years, typically when a baby is switched to formula. Elimination of milk from the diet typically results in symptom remediation within two weeks. Heiner's Syndrome is uncommon, unique to infants, and is usually outgrown in several years. The prevalence of Heiner's Syndrome is unknown (Orphanet 2022).

Eosinophilic Gastroenteritis (EGE)

This is a rare disorder that can involve any portion of the gastrointestinal tract but tends to cause eosinophilic (the roving allergic cell linked to inflammatory damage) invasion in one or more layers of the walls of the stomach and/or intestine. Symptoms depend on the location and layers of the gastrointestinal wall involved and may include heartburn, dysphagia, dyspepsia, abdominal pain, nausea, vomiting, weight loss, bloating, bowel obstruction, and failure to thrive. EGE is a rare condition that affects 8.4 in 100,000 patients and tends to present in children and young adults (Jensen 2016). Having allergies, eczema, and asthma increases the likelihood of developing this disease. Rarely, it can cause ascites (fluid in the abdomen) and pleural effusions (fluid around the lung).

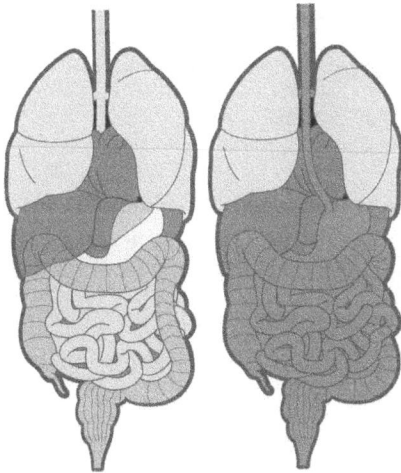

Finding increased levels of IgE and eosinophilia in the blood of patients with typical symptoms is suggestive of EGE. Diagnosis is made by biopsy of affected tissues.

Treatment consists of avoiding foods to which the patient is allergic. Corticosteroids or immunosuppressants can help manage the disease.

Eosinophilic Colitis (EC)

EC is caused by infiltration, injury, and inflammation produced by eosinophils, a type of white blood cell that results in inflammatory damage in the large intes-

Figure 47: Left, normal digestive system. Right, inflammation of EGE starts at the esophagus and affects the entire gastrointestinal tract.

tine. Symptoms include abdominal pain, nausea, vomiting, diarrhea (which may be bloody), weight loss, anemia, fatigue, and malnutrition. Many patients do not determine the triggering agent. As in other eosinophilic disorders, having allergies, eczema, and asthma increases the likelihood of developing this disease. It is very rare, with an estimated prevalence of 10 per 100,000 (Jensen 2016).

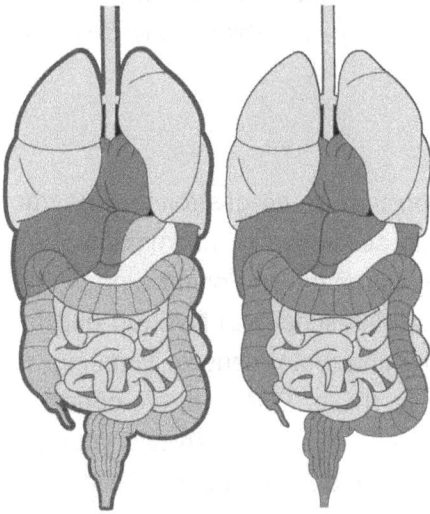

Figure 48: Left, normal digestive system. Right, inflamed large intestine of EC.

Diagnosis occurs with endoscopy, which may show erosions and ulcers, an accompanying biopsy showing eosinophils invading the large intestine, and a colonoscopy with biopsy showing eosinophils causing inflammation. Allergy testing may be helpful to determine which food allergens need to be avoided and prevent excess limitation of the diet. The cornerstone of treatment includes avoidance of food allergen triggers and, if they cannot be identified with testing, use of an elemental diet. To mitigate inflammation, topical and systemic steroids and other anti-inflammatory agents can be used. Iron supplementation and nutritional supplementation may also be required.

Eosinophilic Esophagitis (EoE)

Eosinophilic esophagitis (EoE) is a chronic immunologic condition that causes inflammation of the esophagus, the tube that moves food between the mouth and stomach. EoE can be caused by a Type I IgE-mediated food-specific allergy and/or a Type IV delayed-type allergy caused by damage from immune cells.

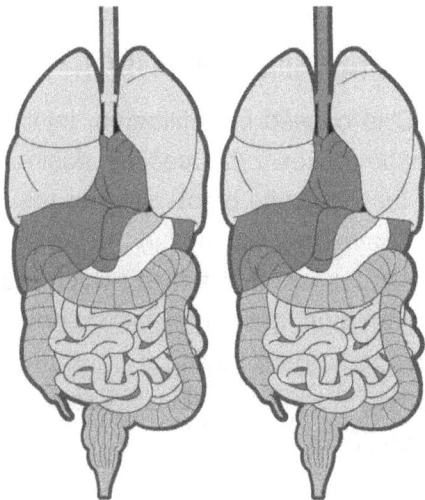

Figure 49: Left, normal digestive system. Right, inflamed esophagus of EoE.

EoE is named after the eosinophils, one type of white blood cell, found in higher than normal numbers in damaged areas of the esophagus. Eosinophils protect us from parasites and certain microbes, but, in this situation, they are the cells damaging the esophagus. When inflammation from eosinophils causes damage to the body, the result is a hypersensitivity disorder.

Eosinophilic esophagitis is a condition caused by inflammation of the esophagus. In young children, it may present as a feeding disorder, vomiting, reflux, and/or abdominal pain, whereas adults may have pain on swallowing and esophageal food catching and impactions. The prevalence of EoE is 1 in 2000 people (ACAAI 2022).

Symptoms

Symptoms of EoE in small children may be as nonspecific as food refusal and failure to thrive or failure to grow at a normal rate. Older children may notice difficulty and pain swallowing, abdominal pain, and vomiting. Teenagers and adults may also have chest pain and heartburn and/or pain and difficulty in swallowing—sometimes to the point it is difficult for them to breathe—especially when eating dry, solid foods. EoE can also cause scarring and subsequent narrowing of the esophagus, further increasing the tendency for food to catch in the throat. Food can become impacted, or stuck without ability to move, and this is an _emergency_.

Diagnosis

The only way to diagnose EoE is through upper endoscopy and biopsy of the esophagus. The criteria for diagnosis of active EoE are 20 eosinophils per high-powered field (of the microscope).

Treatment for EOE

EoE cannot be outgrown: it must be managed. The cornerstone of therapy is monitoring the esophagus for damage. Decrease in damage defines therapy success.

The first part of treatment consists of defining the allergies that are precipitating EoE by environmental and food testing. Because the reaction to food is typically delayed, it is much more challenging to pinpoint the trigger(s).

Six-Food Elimination Diet for EoE

For this reason, the treating physician may opt to have a patient attempt a Six-Food Elimination Diet, which causes remission in nearly 90% of patients. After remission occurs, it is possible to add foods back to the diet one at a time to help delineate which foods were causative and to attempt to ease dietary restrictions. If this is too cumbersome, eliminating just cow's milk, milk and soy, or milk, soy, and wheat may be enough to cause remission but for fewer patients.

The Most Common Food Triggers for EoE

- Cow's milk
- Soy
- Wheat
- Egg
- Peanut and tree nuts
- Seafood (fish and shellfish)

Unfortunately, because EoE is a delayed allergy, it can take weeks to months for the condition to resolve once the trigger food is eliminated from the diet. For this reason, some physicians prefer to perform a food patch testing, in which foods are exposed to the skin for 48 hours, the reaction read, and then a second reading is performed one week after the initial food patch test. Recent studies suggest the usefulness of patch testing for EoE is limited.

If any other foods are positive on testing or are suspected in causing symptoms, fasting and refeeding can be done, but at a much slower pace and with caution, especially if the condition is severe. Refeeding is typically not necessary unless we are not sure whether something is a trigger. I will take the foods most likely to trigger a reaction out of my EoE patient's diet for months (typically at least eight weeks) and then touch base with them to learn how their symptoms are progressing. This decision is based on an extended history of the child's food exposures and reactions.

Once we have gone through the fasting process and I believe we have accurately identified the foods that are creating the problematic reaction, I recommend prolonged and careful avoidance of those foods. After a period of time, I may conduct another endoscopy to double-check that we have effectively addressed every allergen and the esophagus is back to normal. Early in the process, I may refer the patient to a nutritionist or dietician in order to address any missing but important nutrients.

In the meantime, I will address seasonal allergies. In multiple cases, seasonal allergies prevent complete resolution of symptoms in my EoE patients if not addressed. Many patients with EoE note that their symptoms flare seasonally, likely due to the inhalation of environmental allergens. This suggests that environmental allergies should also be tested and treated. In fact, at any given time, I have multiple EoE patients getting allergy shots for environmental allergies solely because they cannot entirely get the relief they need to feel normal unless they address this last trigger of their EoE, the allergens they inhale and then swallow (environmental pollens).

Medication for EoE

Some cases of EoE resolve with proton-pump inhibitors, drugs such as omeprazole, pantoprazole, lansoprazole, rabeprazole, esomeprazole, and dexlansoprazole. This medical condition is then known as proton-pump inhibitor-responsive EoE. Efficacy is validated if biopsy of the esophagus after treatment with a proton-pump inhibitor normalizes the esophagus without additional intervention.

Once elimination of trigger foods and treatment of environmental allergies occurs, the remaining symptoms may be treated with topical steroids. These are the same steroids used by asthma patients until recently. However, instead of inhaling them, this aerosolized liquid is sucked in and swallowed in order to bring the medication to the damaged areas of the esophagus. Corticosteroids kill off eosinophils, eliminating the inflammation and decreasing the damage they cause.

If strictures occur, it may be necessary for the patient to have an esophageal dilation performed to be capable of swallowing food without choking. This is not ideal, however, as every time this procedure occurs, the patient is at risk for esophageal rupture. The more dilation of the esophagus needs to be repeated in the course of a patient's lifetime, the greater the risk to the patient of these complications.

Avoidance through diet is still the best way to go, in my opinion, because long-term steroid use is not ideal and the risks of repeated esophageal dilatation procedures cannot be avoided.

Elemental Diet May Be Used If Other Management Approaches Don't Work

In young children or patients with refractory symptoms, an elemental diet may be used as a last ditch effort to improve refractory symptoms. Nutrition in an elemental diet is entirely dependent on a formula that has no proteins, but only amino acids, sugars, and essential fatty acids. All other solid food is removed from the diet. Because it is not an appetizing diet, as you might imagine, it may need to be administered through a feeding tube. Food is added back to the diet as soon as symptoms resolve in order to normalize the diet as soon as possible. This diet really needs to be supervised by your allergist-immunologist to prevent malnutrition.

Additional medications

Dupilumab (Dupixent) is now indicated for EoE in children 12 years and older. It is now the only FDA-approved biologic medication for eosinophilic esophagitis.

Eczema: The Itch That Rashes

Chapter preview

- Why a compromised skin can increase allergies.
- Why your child's medical history is key to a correct diagnosis.
- How do we test for eczema triggers?
- Multiple management strategies for preserving skin integrity.

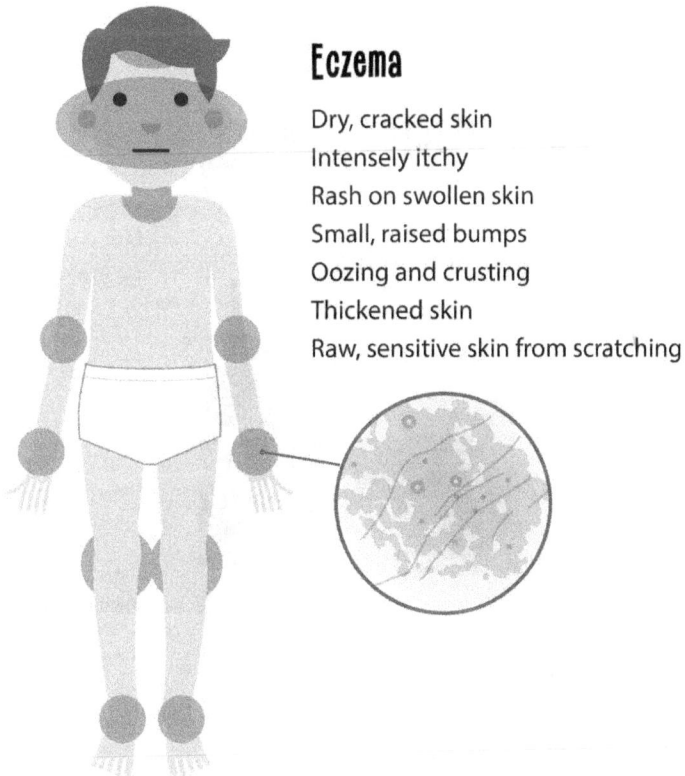

Eczema

Dry, cracked skin
Intensely itchy
Rash on swollen skin
Small, raised bumps
Oozing and crusting
Thickened skin
Raw, sensitive skin from scratching

Figure 50: The rash and symptoms of eczema.

What Is Eczema?

Eczema is one of the most common types of atopic dermatitis and appears as a red, itchy rash or dry, scaly plaques of skin. While it can develop at any age, it usually begins in infancy or young childhood.

What Causes Eczema?

Not everything is known about this condition, but patients with atopic dermatitis (eczema) tend to have a hyperactive immune system that responds to certain triggers with allergic inflammation. Also, patients with atopic dermatitis have an estimated rate of food allergy that is an incredible 35%.

Some patients with atopic dermatitis have a mutation in the connective tissue of the skin that, in healthy skin, is responsible for holding skin cells together and creating a skin barrier. Without an intact barrier, allergens, irritants, bacteria, and viruses can easily enter the area beneath the skin. There, the cells of inflammation react and water is easily lost, making the skin dry and the patient prone to allergy, inflammation, and infection.

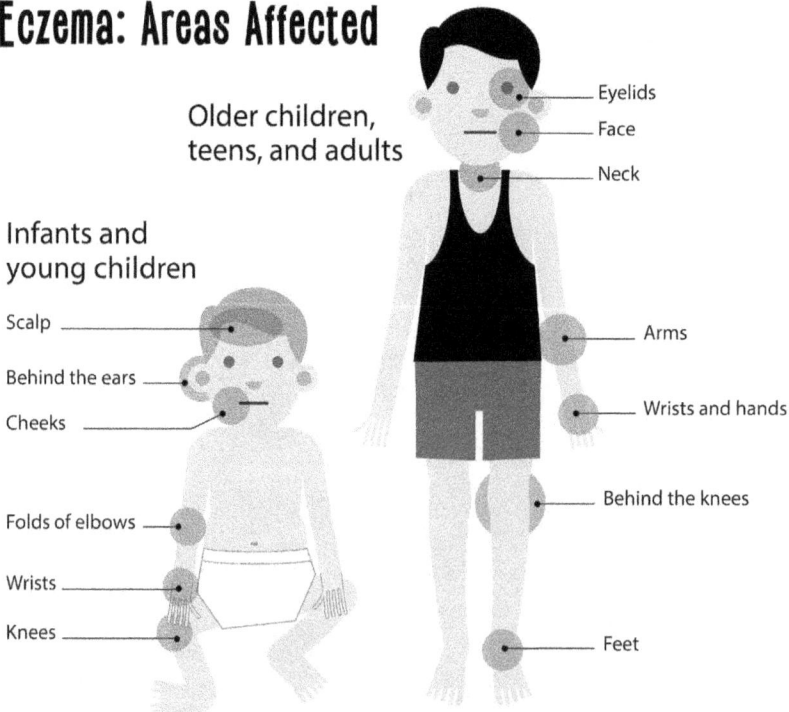

Figure 51: Areas affected by eczema in babies and older children.

Normal Skin
Strong skin barrier

Normal connective tissue holds
adjacent skin cells together
without disruption

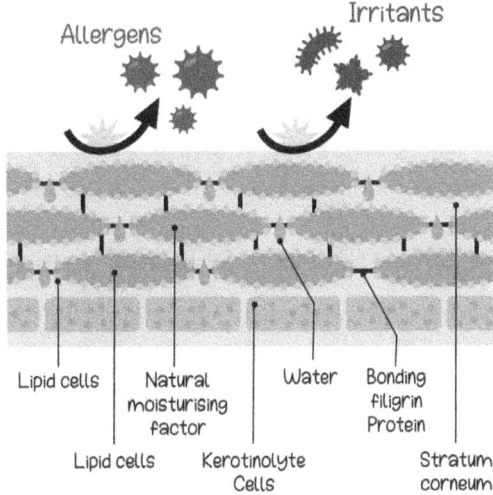

Allergens

Irritants

Lipid cells | Natural moisturising factor | Water | Bonding filigrin Protein

Lipid cells | Kerotinolyte Cells | Stratum corneum

Skin with Eczema
Weakened skin barrier

Entry of allergens, bacteria, yeast,
mold, and irritants to the layer underneath
the skin, results in inflammation.

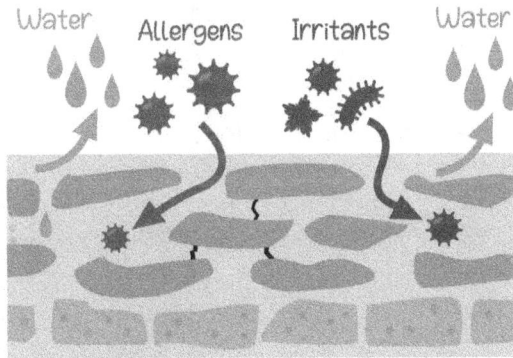

Water

Allergens

Irritants

Water

Loss of water affects
skin cells and cellular
function and making
them more fragile

Mutated connective tissue
causes a dysfunctional,
fragile barrier between
skin cells.

Figure 52: Normal skin with its normal connective tissue has an intact skin barrier and is well hydrated. It can keep water in and allergens, pathogens, and irritants out. Eczematous skin has deformed connective tissue, leading to a deformed skin barrier, water loss, and penetration of allergens, pathogens, and irritants.

A Compromised Skin Barrier Invites Allergens Into the Body

Patients with atopic dermatitis live with higher rates of food allergy and environmental allergy and are more likely to develop asthma, due to dysfunction of their protective skin barrier. Further, patients with untreated atopic dermatitis have among the highest rate of increase of allergies. This means if allergy tests were first conducted on a patient with atopic dermatitis at age two and then again at age twenty, the patient would be very likely to have a far greater increase in the number of additional allergies than a patient without atopic dermatitis. Patients with atopic dermatitis also have higher rates of anxiety and depression, thought to be due to a greatly impaired quality of life.

Skin Testing May Help Identify Your Child's Allergic Triggers

All methods of skin testing can be challenging in patients with eczema and other conditions in which the skin is highly inflamed. Therefore, if patient history can point to likely food triggers, that is an ideal place to begin the process.

In eczema patients, allergic reactions are most commonly immediate, starting within minutes of exposure to the trigger, but they can also be delayed and literally not affect the skin for weeks. For this reason, skin prick testing for food and environmental allergies can help identify immediate-type allergy triggers, while patch testing may help identify delayed allergies. Following skin testing, a fasting and refeeding strategy can help validate the findings of the skin tests and theories based on patient history.

Below is a list of triggers that make eczema worse:

- Allergies (food) - The most common foods that contribute to eczema are milk, wheat, soy, egg, nut, tree nut, fish, shellfish, and sesame
- Allergies (environmental)
- Harmful skin bacteria and skin infections
- Chemicals
- Sun, sweat, and sunscreen
- Hot water
- Stress
- Scratchy or occlusive clothing

How Do I Manage My Atopic Dermatitis?

Skin Hydration and Care

The first and most important part of atopic dermatitis management is learning proper skin hydration techniques. The skin is hydrated to remove bacteria and irritants and to help seal in moisture, enhance the skin barrier, and protect it from irritants and allergens. Hydration techniques help bolster the skin's protective layer. Skin infections and bacterial carriage on the skin should be controlled, as both further damage fragile eczematous skin.

Avoid Dehydration of Your Child's Skin

- Hot water can be irritating and strip precious oil from eczematous skin.
  - o Use cool to lukewarm rather than hot water.
  - o Rather than rubbing your child dry after a shower or bath, gently pat skin dry and apply a moisturizing, hypoallergenic cream to help lock in moisture and prevent precious skin oils from being wiped away.
- Weather changes can also be problematic, due to drying of skin. During dry weather, step up your game and be mindful of skin hydration.
- Sun, heat, and dryness can lead to dehydration of already-fragile skin. Dehydration deforms skin cells and makes them more fragile, increasing the rash of eczema.
- Sunscreen sensitivity can be tested with patch testing, but mineral versions of sunscreens like zinc oxide and titanium dioxide are generally better for sensitive skin than chemical sunscreen. Remaining in the shade and staying cool can also minimize irritation.
- Stress is an enormous trigger for eczema. Illness and stress hormones can tip the delicate balance of the immune system, which is already dysfunctional in eczema patients. The itch habit is increased, which may be a self-soothing technique for some patients. This makes the rash even worse.

Habit Scratching

The importance of "habit scratching" cannot be understated. It is a major problem in children with eczema. Not long ago, I helped a child completely alleviate his eczema. However, long after the rash was gone and the child denied being "itchy," I would catch him scratching during the exam. I thought, *If I am catching this poor child scratching during my 15-20 minute visit with him, he has to be scratching himself at home.*

His mom and I had to come up with multiple ways to help him stop habit scratching and damaging his skin. Some suggestions I made (and I think it took all of them for his mom to solve the problem) were: distracting him, keeping his hands busy, changing the "itch" habit into an "apply the moisturizing cream" habit, bringing the scratching to his attention, wearing bulky gloves that make scratching harder to do and gentler, and observing and avoiding any situations or exposures that increased the itch (like stress).

Avoid Allergic Triggers

The second most important treatment for eczema is avoidance of food allergens that increase the rash. Food triggers should be carefully identified and then eliminated from the diet.

The third most important treatment for eczema is avoidance of environmental allergens. Environmental allergies should be tested, identified, and avoided whenever possible. Those environmental pollen and other allergens that cannot be avoided, such as mold and pet dander, are best treated by your child's allergist-immunologist with allergy shots (allergen immunotherapy), which pivots the immune reaction to a less allergic, more neutral response.

Avoid Contact with Chemicals That Irritate Skin

Knowing that anything irritating to the skin can trigger eczema, it's very important for patients with eczema or any type of atopic dermatitis to avoid contact with chemicals. My recommendations include:

- Avoid skin contact with chemicals, including household cleaners.
- Wear cotton-lined gloves while cleaning.
- Avoid unnecessary skin exposure and inhalation of air fresheners, perfumes, and scented candles.
- Use moisturizing and hypoallergenic skin care products whenever possible. Avoid the use of abrasive skin cleansers and exfoliators that strip the oil from and mechanically damage the skin.
- Attempt to use hypoallergenic soaps, shampoos, detergents, and laundry products whenever possible. Bear in mind that "hypoallergenic" does not mean non-allergenic; less than 1 in 100 patients develop reactions to hypoallergenic substances, but that number is definitely not zero. However, hypoallergenic and Free & Clear products with neutral pH are less likely to be problematic. If there is a need to determine which product is causing your child's symptoms, patch testing can also be used to identify the allergenic substance.
- Loose cotton clothes are best for sensitive skin. Synthetic materials like polyester can retain sweat and heat and irritate the skin, but even natural fibers like wool may irritate the skin.
- Avoid dry cleaning your child's clothes. Rather, use wrinkle-free/perma-press clothes. Before wearing, wash new clothes with Free & Clear laundry products to remove the fabric finishing chemicals. If skin irritation still occurs, consider allergy patch testing for Free & Clear detergents and fabric softeners.

◆ ◆ ◆

Shortly after birth, we noticed that my son, Alex, had some intense eczema as well as severe digestive issues: fussiness, abdominal distention, and diarrhea. I took him off cow's milk, which helped, but clearly was not the complete answer. I removed soy from his diet too and that did the trick—his symptoms completely resolved. Once every year, I would try to add milk and soy back into his diet and his symptoms would return. Then, when he was about seven years old, he was able to successfully consume milk and soy and we've never looked back. I was so happy, since my entire top refrigerator shelf had different milks for everyone in the family. Now we are down to just three different milks (learn more about lactose intolerance in Chapter 20).

Alex has been a work in progress and his many sensitivities have evolved over the years. First, I had to work with his food allergy. Then I focused on skin hydration—we only used the gentlest of hydrating cleansers in the shower.

Recently, I retested his environmental allergies. Now, I will tell you that a few years ago one of his doctors did a blood allergy panel that came out completely negative—the test showed he wasn't allergic to any substance tested. However, this time, only a few years later, we tried an allergy skin test. By the end of the exam, he was in tears because he had so many large hives. The majority of the tests were *positive*—he was allergic to a good majority of grass, trees, weeds, and ragweed on the test. Well, no wonder he kept having issues!

With this new information, I've managed to slow the crawl of his allergies and eczema. I forgot to mention his reactive airway, which, thankfully, has never developed into asthma. I do not know if he would have become asthmatic if I had not been so aggressive in taking care of him, but I am very glad that I was able to and did.

In case you think that just because I am an allergist-immunologist this was a quick and easy path, I want to reassure you that it was not. There were times when his symptoms were unbearable and kept him up at night. He was a trooper and, piece by piece, we solved the puzzle of his allergies. From time to time, they still create issues (he is now a teenager) but they are not nearly as distracting and problematic as when he was a baby.

◆ ◆ ◆

How Is Atopic Dermatitis Treated by Allergist-Immunologists?

Hydrate to Improve the Skin Barrier

Skin hydration is the foundation of eczema care; some patients' symptoms can be controlled with skin hydration alone. It is estimated that with hydration techniques alone, the rate of increase of allergies in eczema patients is reduced by 50%.

Hydration creates, protects, and increases the elasticity of the skin barrier. This reduces water loss and minimizes the penetration of inflammatory allergens that could trigger the allergy cells underneath the skin. Both dehydration and intrusion of allergens escalate the damage.

Recommended: Four levels of hydration

There are four levels of hydration, the first being the most basic for all patients with eczema, the second intended for easily controlled eczema, the third for moderate to severe eczema, and the fourth for flares of eczema.

1. Daily hydration for all patients with atopic dermatitis:

Use an ultra-gentle hydrating wash with ceramides, pat skin dry (don't rub), and apply a moisturizing cream formulated for eczema.

2. Hydration for mild, persistent eczema:

a. To bathe, use an ultra-gentle hydrating wash with ceramides on moist skin. Pat dry; do not rub dry.
b. Apply a thin layer of extra-virgin olive oil. A drop is all that is frequently necessary. Your child does not need to look like a salad.
c. Apply a thin layer of moisturizing cream with ceramides.
d. Apply a thin layer of petroleum jelly.
e. Wrap affected extremities with cotton gauze. When severely affected, consider wrapping with plastic wrap (not for a small child).
f. Cover with "hydrating pajamas" (see instructions later in this chapter or leave gauze or plastic wrap in place, if adult or older child).
g. Leave on for 20 minutes.
h. Wipe off excess.
i. When rash subsides, use only moisturizing cream with ceramides in areas typically affected.

3. Bleach bath instructions for patients with moderate to severe persistent eczema:

As intimidating as a bleach bath may sound, it's equivalent to swimming in a chlorinated pool, except you control the amount of chlorination. I assure you (from experience), when performed properly, it is safe and effective. As much work as it is, it can provide a lot of relief (although I have to admit, I am glad that we only have to perform step 1 now, and only as needed at that).

   a. Fill a tub for a normal bath (about 40 gallons) with lukewarm water. Never use or allow skin to come into contact with undiluted bleach.
   b. Place one-quarter to one-half cup of common liquid bleach into the bath water. Before using bleach, read the label to check that the concentration of bleach (sodium hypochlorite 6% should be listed on the contents label without any other chemicals).
   c. Mix the bleach in the water. Just to reassure you, this is just a little stronger than appropriately chlorinated pool water.
   d. Test that the bleach water is thoroughly mixed.
   e. Soak in the chlorinated water for about 10-20 minutes.
   f. Thoroughly rinse the skin clear with clean, lukewarm water.
   g. Pat dry gently, do not rub.
   h. Apply prescribed moisturizing cream or medication as soon as possible.
   i. This may be repeated two to three times per week, but if used more frequently, this treatment may dry the skin. Be careful about using bleach baths if there are many breaks in your child's skin, as it may be irritating or even painful. Monitor results because if it is too drying, it is advisable to use bleach baths less frequently.

Always be cautious around bleach and a tub of water and your child. Maintain control of the bleach bottle. Make sure the bleach is only sodium hypochlorite at 6%. Add one-fourth to one-half cup bleach to the tub of water, mix thoroughly, then place the bleach container in a safe area away from your child. As drownings can happen in an inch of water and accidents like slipping and falling can occur, it is imperative to be present during this entire process from the time the tub is being filled with water until the tub is completely drained after the bath.

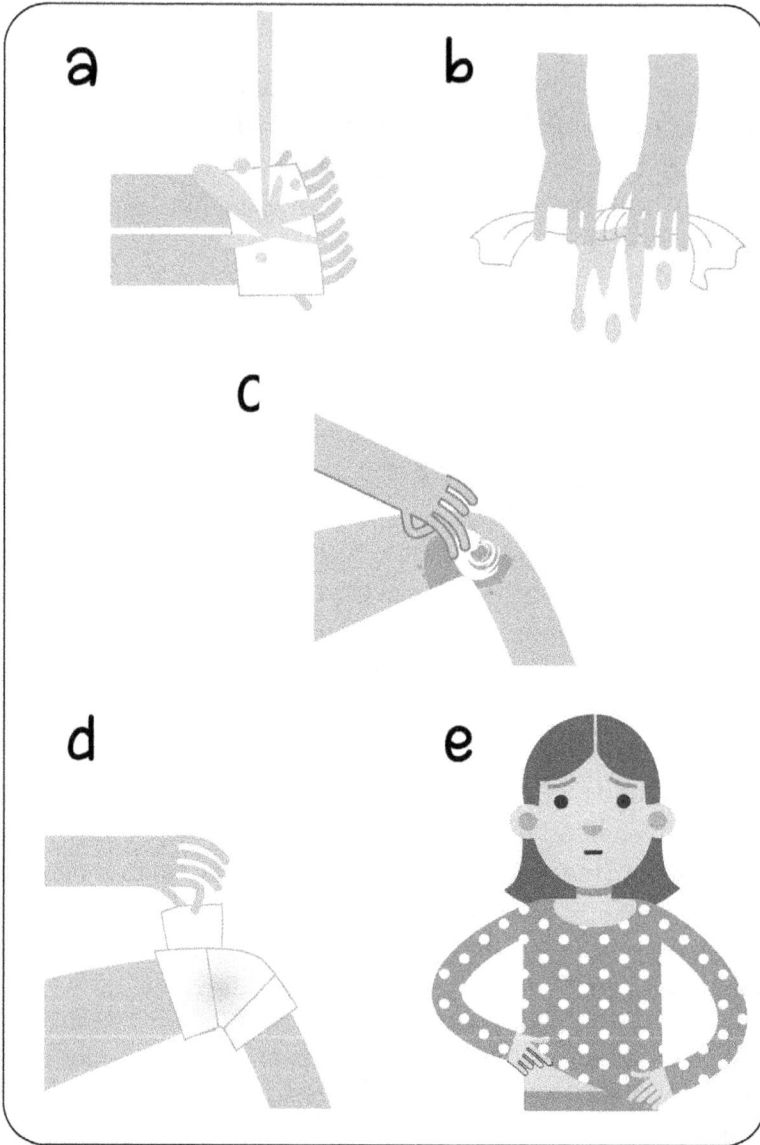

Figure 53: Below are instructions for each step of the wet to dry wrap treatment.

4. Wet to dry wrap for severe eczema and eczema flares:

This treatment works best after bathing or moisturizing and medicating. It should only be performed under the supervision of your child's allergist-immunologist.

a. Soak a roll of clean cotton gauze briefly in lukewarm water.
b. Wring out the roll of gauze as hard as possible so it is barely damp.
c. Apply prescription topical steroid to your child's skin as recommended by your child's allergist-immunologist.

d. Wrap affected areas with the damp gauze.

e. Wrap the dry areas with dry gauze. Put on cotton gloves and socks, if desired. Then put on a snug layer of dry, nighttime clothing over both wet and dry wraps so they remain undisturbed and in place overnight.

As an alternative for younger children, a snugger set of pajamas with a long-sleeved shirt and long pants can be used for the wet layer and a looser set that can fit over the wet layer can be used for the dry layer.

Test to Identify Allergic Triggers

Allergy testing for food and environmental allergies and patch testing for chemical allergy are the two quickest, easiest, and most accurate tests when performed by a board-certified allergist-immunologist. To briefly recap allergy skin testing, a small amount of food, pollen, pet dander, mold, or insect extract is placed just underneath the skin in the layer above that contains the master allergic cells (see Chapter 3 for a more detailed explanation). If recognized, the allergic cell releases histamine, which causes leakage and dilation of the blood vessel(s) under the skin to form a hive. No reaction occurs in areas that are not recognized by the allergy cells. This type of testing is used for allergies that cause an immediate reaction.

To summarize, in the patch testing process, chemicals in various dilutions are placed in contact with the skin for a prolonged time and then the irritation or allergic inflammation is read and interpreted. This testing is best for delayed-type allergy, or that which takes time to develop (see Chapter 14 for a more detailed explanation).

Eliminate the Itch

Allergists have nicknamed eczema "the itch that rashes" and call the flares caused by the trauma of itching the "itch-scratch cycle." The frail skin of the eczema sufferer is damaged by this usually minor trauma. Itching also has a huge effect on sleep and stress for eczema patients, worsening their already compromised quality of life.

The solution is to avoid food, environmental, and chemical triggers and start allergy shots for unavoidable environmental allergens. Any remaining itch should be treated with antihistamines and anti-leukotrienes.

Reduce Inflammation

Depending on the severity and acuity, atopic dermatitis is treated with topical steroids, antibiotics, phototherapy, biologics, and immunosuppressants to control inflammation that cannot be managed in other ways.

Topical steroids have been the mainstay of treatment until recently. These should be used under an allergist-immunologist's supervision, as they have many side effects, including thinned skin and infections. One significant advantage of topical steroids is that they tend to be fast-acting. Sensitive areas such as the eyelids, face, and genitals should be avoided.

Steroids are available in multiple strengths. Stronger steroids are used for a shorter period of time during flares and on thicker areas of skin. Once controlled, the strength is reduced.

Because regular use can result in "steroid flare"—a condition in which withdrawal of a steroid results in the eczema rash worsening significantly—it is advised, once the steroid strength is reduced and the rash controlled, that the medication be tapered rather than stopped abruptly.

For example, if the steroid triamcinolone was used twice daily for two weeks and the rash is gone, the triamcinolone should then be used once daily for one week, every other day for one week, and twice weekly for one week. If at any time the rash becomes worse, return to the last application schedule in which control was achieved and slow or stop the taper.

Topical calcineurin inhibitors, such as tacrolimus (Protopic) and pimecrolimus (Elidel) help control eczema and are particularly helpful for sensitive areas like the face. They may require a month or more to take effect and need to be used regularly to work completely.

Crisaborole (Eucrisa) is a topical phosphodiesterase-4 (an enzyme that increases inflammation) inhibitor that controls activation of immune cells and the resulting inflammation in the skin. It may require a month or more to take effect and needs to be used regularly to be effective.

Dupilumab (Dupixent) is the first biologic agent to be FDA-approved for atopic dermatitis. Dupixent targets the immune system cells that create the inflammation of eczema. Regular use reduces inflammation, itch, redness, and rash. Dupixent is a prescribed drug for use in patients six years old and older that have moderate to severe atopic dermatitis.

In extremely difficult eczema cases, drugs that suppress the immune system such as methotrexate, mycophenolate, and cyclosporine are used. These drugs are not FDA-approved for this purpose (they are FDA approved for other conditions) but have been used successfully before we found adequate treatment for atopic dermatitis. Many side effects are possible and therefore, they must be prescribed by physicians and carefully monitored.

Barrier Maintenance

The first step to barrier maintenance is over-the-counter creams and emollients with ceramides. If these products are not helpful, your child's allergist-immunologist may try prescription creams. These creams supply the lipids and ceramides from fats, oils, and waxes that eczema patients typically lack.

Recommendations to Minimize Stress

Patients with chronic eczema have among the highest rates of anxiety and depression when compared with patients with other severe and chronic illnesses, yet the immune system does not work properly when under stress. Because of this, it is my recommendation that stress be addressed as well.

Here are some suggestions to decrease stress:

- Make sleep a priority.
- Eat healthy meals regularly.
- Distract your child with activities he/she enjoys and that require concentration, like puzzles.
- Be gentle on yourself and your child: this is not your fault, nor is it his/hers.
- Don't nag about scratching. Instead, help them replace the behavior with a healthier habit, such as applying moisturizer every time they feel like scratching.
- Try relaxation techniques like yoga, meditation, and prayer.
- Exercise. This releases hormones that protect us, relax us, and make us feel better. The release of "feel good" hormones during exercise is known as "runner's high."
- Laugh. Comedy shows, funny movies, and funny people are great stress relievers.
- Have your child call a friend and connect with others. It is widely believed that as a society, we have lost so much connection with other people, and this is an incredible source of anxiety, depression, depersonalization, and dehumanization.
- Journal: have your child write about his/her feelings.
- Be creative: try having your child draw, color, paint, play music, and/or listen to relaxing music.
- Let your child take time for himself/herself.
- Try (and this is hard) not to dwell on the negative and don't let your child dwell. Teach your child to recognize what he/she is doing, try to change thoughts or journal about how he/she could change. Understand that it is natural to "go negative," as this is a survival mechanism. After all, the lamb that thought the lion would treat her well probably did not last as long as the one that was wary and anxious in his presence.
- Be positive and try to encourage positivity in your child. Challenge your child to name three good events of the day. Have them write them in a journal and reread them from time to time; this will reinforce positive thinking.

- Ask your child to give someone a compliment. This not only makes the person they compliment feel good, it increases positive feelings toward your child.
- Show your child how to help others. Working at a charitable event for a good cause is known to increase the "feel good" hormones. This response has been called "helper's high."
- Find a support group. Bring your child and encourage them to talk it out with people that understand what he/she is going through.
- Get professional help to cope with excess worry or negative thinking, especially if his/her thoughts are extreme or involve self-harm or harming others.

Part 5: Food Intolerance

Chapter 20

Ready to Rumble:
Food Intolerance and Irritable Bowel Syndrome

Chapter Preview

- Learn the definitions of food intolerance and irritable bowel syndrome (IBS).
- How are food intolerances diagnosed and treated?
- How is irritable bowel syndrome diagnosed and treated?
- What is a FODMAP and how does it play a role in treatment?

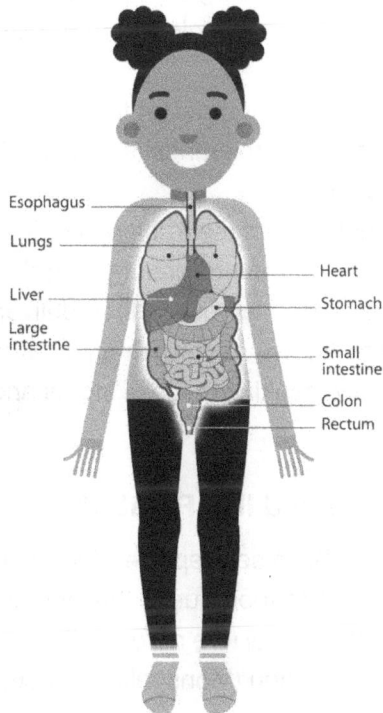

Figure 54: Normal gastrointestinal system.

What Is Irritable Bowel Syndrome? (IBS)

IBS is a very common disorder of the intestines that causes abdominal pain, gas, bloating, and is either diarrhea-predominant (IBS-D), constipation-dominant (IBS-C), or vacillates between both (IBS-M). The exact cause is not known but is likely multifactorial.

Currently, one of the leading theories is that IBS "include[s] the presence of visceral hypersensitivity, gut dysmotility, mucosal inflammation, and changes in the makeup of the intestinal microbiota" (Crowe 2019).

Food intolerance may cause a flare of IBS or may be one of the symptoms, as most patients with IBS have food intolerance. Therefore, addressing it is considered one of the first steps in treatment.

What Is Food Intolerance?

Food intolerance presents as uncomfortable symptoms that arise after eating specific foods. The typical symptom pattern is loose stools to diarrhea, abdominal pain, bloating, distention, and altered motility that occurs shortly after eating that specific food. Unlike anaphylaxis, food intolerance does not cause other signs of immediate allergy such as shortness of breath, wheezing, chest tightness, swelling of the throat or tongue, flushing, or hives. Further, allergenic foods tend to fit a common pattern—the foods that most commonly cause allergic symptoms are milk, egg, fish, shellfish, peanuts, tree nuts, soy, and wheat.

In contrast, intolerant foods may or may not fit that pattern. While there may be a variety of causes, many times food intolerance is an inability to digest a substance in the amount that was consumed.

The most common example is lactose intolerance, in which the person affected does not make enough lactase enzyme to break down the lactose in dairy products to enable its absorption. Undigested lactose is then delivered to the intestine, where bacteria digest it in a process known as fermentation, which consists of fluid shifts and intestinal irritation, typically resulting in loose stools and gas production that may cause bloating and pain.

How Are Food Intolerance and IBS Related?

Up to 70% of patients with IBS have self-reported food intolerance.

Many believe they are allergic to food due to the increase in symptoms they experience after eating. However, the actual rate of food allergy amongst patients with IBS parallels that of the general population (Monsbakken 2006).

There are other food intolerances, as we shall discuss later in this chapter, that are completely unrelated to IBS. Therefore, most patients with IBS have a food intolerance but not all food intolerance is a result of IBS.

LACTOSE INTOLERANCE
SYMPTOMS

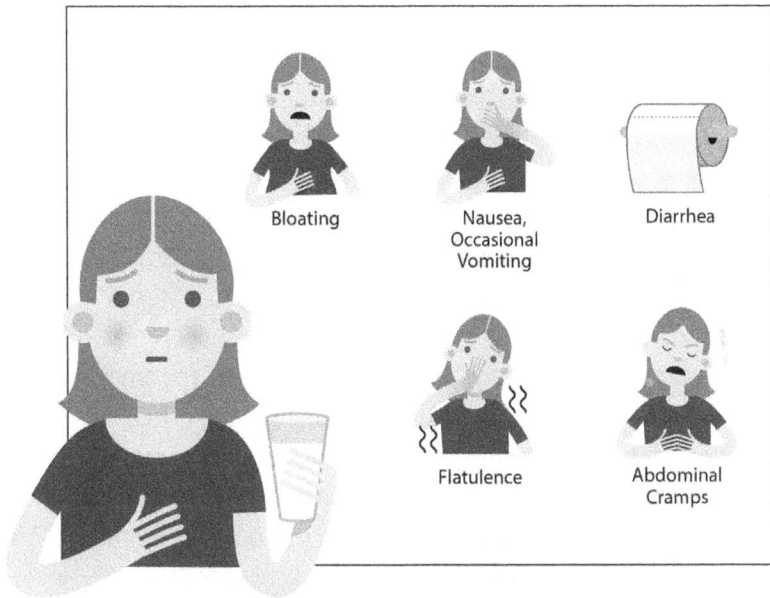

Bloating

Nausea, Occasional Vomiting

Diarrhea

Flatulence

Abdominal Cramps

LACTOSE INTOLERANCE
MANAGEMENT

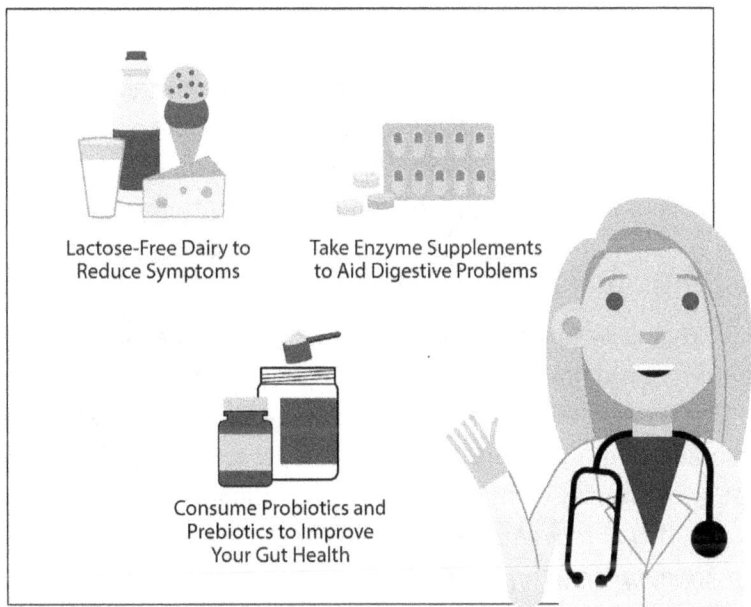

Lactose-Free Dairy to Reduce Symptoms

Take Enzyme Supplements to Aid Digestive Problems

Consume Probiotics and Prebiotics to Improve Your Gut Health

Figure 55: Symptoms and management strategies for lactose intolerance.

How Is Food Intolerance Diagnosed?

First, be aware of the presence or absence of other gastrointestinal issues. If any of the above warning signs are occurring or if your child has other symptoms, I recommend further evaluation, probably with a gastroenterologist.

Second, a thorough patient history questionnaire can help your child's allergist-immunologist assess whether or not he/she has a food intolerance. Organize your thoughts about your child's symptoms ahead of time and then bring your answers to your physician. However, a questionnaire is an adjunct and not a substitute for a thorough history, physical exam, and evaluation by a family physician/pediatrician, allergist-immunologist, and/or dietician/nutritionist. It is not designed to be a stand-alone diagnostic tool.

Third, and depending on the age of the patient, I may recommend a limited time trial (of four to six weeks, never more than six) using a "low FODMAP diet" (see below), followed by a rechallenge using one FODMAP at a time to determine their trigger FODMAP(s), then maintaining a lower (but not zero) intake of the triggering FODMAP. In younger children, normalizing the diet in terms of pediatric dietary guidelines—that is, avoiding excessive fruit, including fruit juice and dried fruit, wheat, including bread and snack foods, and dairy, including milk and yogurt. I agree with Monash University that a restrictive diet should be a last resort for a child (Monash email communication, November 2022; Collins 2020).

Fourth and finally, in teenagers (and adults), I recommend consumption of the FODMAP or FODMAPs (one at a time at various/varying doses over the course of the following four to six weeks) to fine-tune your comfortable "dose" or dose range. At this point, you can use FODMAP tables from reliable sources if the FODMAP app does not include all the foods in your child's diet to help guide the amount of food that your child can consume without triggering his/her symptoms.

How Is IBS Diagnosed?

There is no definitive test to diagnose IBS. However, the Rome IV criteria is considered the current standard and is used in research studies to evaluate patients for IBS. The Rome IV criteria for IBS requires that a patient be symptomatic for at least six months and that abdominal pain and at least two of the following symptoms are present at least one day each week of the previous three months: abdominal pain associated with bowel movements, a change in frequency of bowel movements, and a change in appearance of bowel movements. It is essential that other potential causes of these symptoms be ruled out as well, which is why it is best to seek advice from an experienced physician if IBS is suspected.

Treatment of Food Intolerance Starts Identification of the Trigger

The initial treatment of food intolerance is identifying and avoiding the problematic foods. In some cases, that may be dairy products alone or wheat alone. If that is known, keeping consumption below the threshold that flares your child's symptoms may be all that is needed. If not, using a FODMAP diet may be useful.

What Is a FODMAP?

FODMAP was designed to address symptoms of IBS. It is my first recommendation for treating IBS. The typical problem foods are usually sugars, collectively known as FODMAPs (*Fermentable Oligosaccharides, D-saccharides, Monosaccharides and Polyols*). More familiar names of some of these sugars are fructose, fructans, galacto-oligosaccharides (GOS), and polyols such as sorbitol and mannitol.

What Impact Do FODMAPs Have on the Body?

Have you ever noticed that sugar-free candy has a warning on the package similar to this one? *Excess consumption may cause stomach upset or have a laxative effect.*

The reason for the warning is this: the FODMAPs and artificial sweeteners in sugar-free candy are literally indigestible and cause significant symptoms of intolerance—abdominal pain, bloating and distention, and loose stools. The result? Vast numbers of people are eating FODMAPS without understanding that excess consumption of FODMAPs, such as those present in artificial sweeteners and processed foods, are causing their pain and suffering and driving them to seek help from allergist-immunologists like me, thinking that their symptoms and suffering must be due to a food allergy.

Further, food investigators say that sugar alcohols like sorbitol and mannitol are formulated specifically to drive over-consumption. While the food may be tasty, these artificial sweeteners do not satisfy the appetite, making it easy for consumers to overeat. Further, a person with a sweet tooth like me can be persuaded that because the calorie count is low and the food essentially passes through the digestive system without absorption and therefore without calories. These food manufacturers want you to believe there is no downside to overeating sugar-free products so that you will continue to buy them and your child will continue to overeat them, but this is clearly not the case.

How Does the FODMAP Diet Work and Where Do I Find It?

My recommendation is to use the Monash University FODMAP diet app (https://www.monashfodmap.com/). Once inside the app, you will find lists of food groups, such as vegetables, fruits, and breads.

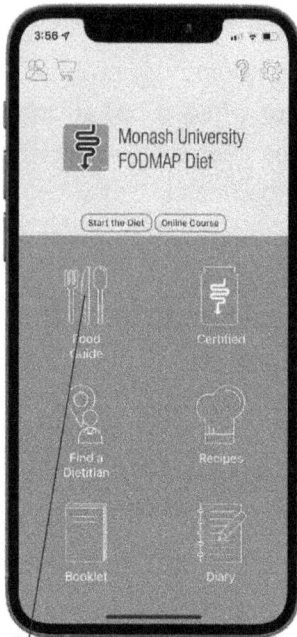

STEP 1

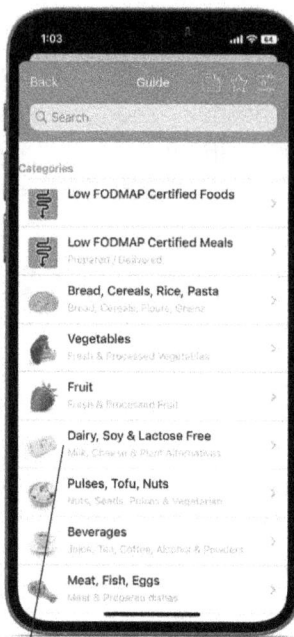

STEP 2

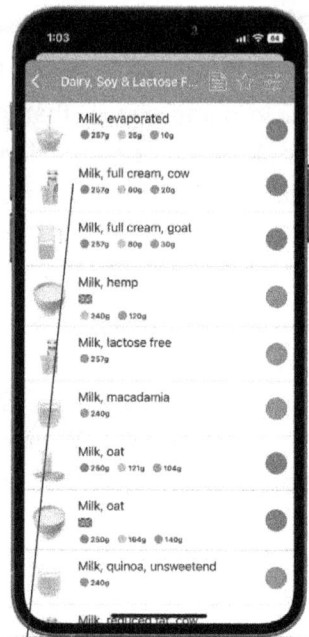

STEP 3a

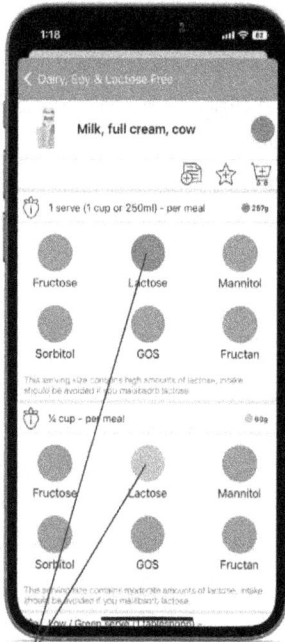

STEP 3b

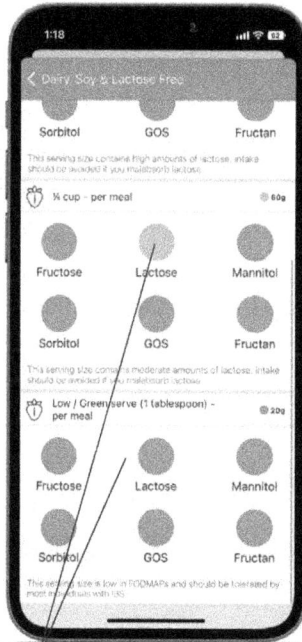

STEP 3c

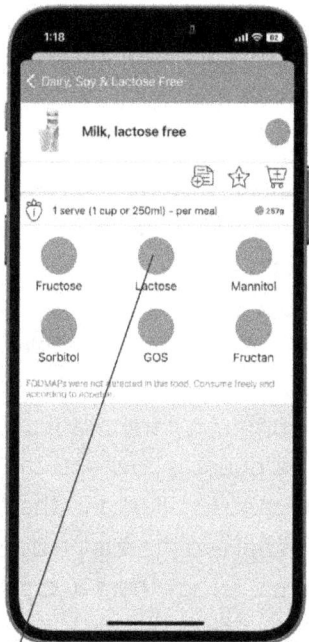

STEP 3d

Figure 56: Source: Department of Gastroenterology, Monash University. Images reproduced with permission from Monash University (monashfodmap.com). Download the Monash University FODMAP Diet App for a comprehensive food guide containing the FODMAP ratings and serving sizes for hundreds of different foods and beverages. Available on iOS and Android.

Instructions for FODMAP App

Step 1: Open the food guide.

Step 2: Find the food group you are looking for. In this illustration, we are searching for milk. This would be found in the "Dairy, Soy, and Lactose-Free" category. Find milk or search for milk in the search bar at the top.

Step 3a: Open the milk page and look at the colored dots; they indicate the amount of lactose in each serving size.

Step 3b and c: You will see that while the other five FODMAPs—fructose, mannitol, sorbitol, GOS, and fructan—are green, the lactose dot changes from red to yellow to green according to the serving size.

One cup of full cream milk (250 ml) = 257 grams. The lactose dot is red, indicating a high amount of lactose.

One-fourth cup of full cream milk = 60 grams. The lactose dot is amber, indicating a moderate amount of lactose.

One tablespoon of full cream milk = 20 grams. The lactose dot is green, indicating a low amount of lactose.

Step 3d: Review a different dairy product, lactose-free milk:

One cup of lactose-free milk (250 ml) = 257 grams. The lactose dot is green, indicating a low amount of lactose.

A low FODMAP diet is a short-term reduction (two to six weeks) in all FODMAPs under the supervision of a nutritionist, dietician, or physician. A process of re-challenging the specific FODMAPs commences when the overseeing nutritionist, dietician, or physician requests reintroduction of the FODMAPs at higher levels. A diet is then adapted to the patient after interpreting and re-challenging, if necessary. The goal is to reintroduce foods based on response and only to restrict those that trigger symptoms.

I emphasize that, due to the potential for malnutrition, a low FODMAP diet should be done under the direct care of your child's nutritionist, dietician, or physician. For younger children, as previously mentioned, the gentle FODMAP diet is more appropriate.

What are the warning signs your symptoms could be something more dangerous?

Although food intolerance is just that—an inability to comfortably eat all of a typical portion of a food—some symptoms are considered "red flags," a warning that something more ominous is going on than food intolerance. If the following symptoms start over the age of 50 and are severe and worsening, the patient is advised to review them with his/her primary care physician:

Symptoms that may be warning signs: unexplained weight loss, nocturnal diarrhea, rectal bleeding, bloody or black stools, or iron-deficiency anemia. Patients who have family members with colon cancer, celiac disease, or inflammatory bowel disease (like Crohn's or ulcerative colitis) should disclose this to their physician as well.

Your Child's Microbiome

The microbiome has become a trendy and popular topic in modern medicine. The microbiome is a collection of bacteria and other microbes that inhabit various areas of the body, and "talk" via various cell signals and chemical substances. These chemical substances can affect our physiology and metabolism in a good way or a bad way. Those microbes that affect our metabolism in a positive way are regarded as beneficial. Those that affect our metabolism in a negative way are regarded as problematic or even disease-causing. Researchers studying the gut of patients with inflammatory bowel disease* (IBD), a very serious, potentially life-threatening form of gut inflammation, noted that when their patients were fed good microbes in the form of a probiotic, their condition improved. We've now learned that many areas of the body have a microbiome and that they even talk to each other.

*Do not confuse IBD with irritable bowel syndrome (IBS), which can be miserable but is not life-threatening.

What Is the Role of Probiotics in IBS, Food Allergies, and Food Intolerance?

There are differences in the microbiome of the gut of an unaffected patient and one who has IBS, food allergy, or food intolerance. There have been a limited number of studies that have shown success in probiotic supplementation allaying the symptoms of IBS as well as modifying the development of food allergies and intolerance. While use of probiotics for these conditions is nowhere near being ready for prime time, it is hopeful that one day our knowledge of the microbiome will increase enough that we can confidently endorse its use to prevent and possibly treat these conditions (Pimentel 2020; Nance 2020; Caminero 2019).

If standard, refrigerated probiotics are not helpful, consider purchasing from a company that checks your child's current profile of bacteria (with a stool culture) and creates a custom probiotic for him/her, rather than a one-size-fits-all probiotic. Also, if symptoms seem to worsen when he/she starts the probiotic, try cutting the dose for a while and then slowly increase it. Be careful to avoid probiotics sold off in a non-refrigerated area of the store. While there can be no guarantees regarding the store's treatment of these products before or after they are placed on the shelf or how they are transported, more of the bacteria will survive if they are handled carefully.

If your child's probiotics are powdered or in capsule form, just add it to a non-carbonated fruit juice (carbonation kills the bacteria), mix, and drink. Start with a quarter-dose or a half-dose and slowly increase. If your child's probiotic supplier doesn't monitor your child's progress and adjust your child's probiotic as you go, I recommend that you alternate probiotics with different varieties of bacteria to increase your child's gut microbiome diversity. If your child's probiotic gives him/her gastrointestinal side effects, start at a lower amount and increase slowly.

My favorite type of probiotic company tailors a probiotic for your child by taking a stool sample and analyzing the microbiome. It evaluates beneficial and potentially harmful microbes and evaluates the diversity of the microbiome. It then seeks to dilute the potentially harmful microbes and increase the beneficial microbes as well as the diversity of the gut microbiome. This company ensures that its product arrives at your doorstep with as many viable bacteria as possible. Best of all, they communicate with their clients to ensure benefit.

What Is the Role of Food Allergies in IBS?

Technically speaking, these are two separate entities. However, patients can have food allergies and IBS. Food allergies already limit the diet. IBS limits the diet further. Unfortunately, IBS makes patients feel so uncomfortable after they eat that they begin to fixate about eating and food in general.

If this is the case with your child, get help from an experienced dietician, nutritionist, or physician.

What Is the Role of Food Allergy Testing in IBS?

IBS issues are enhanced by food intolerance and possibly inflammation, not necessarily food allergy. In many patients with gut issues, especially those patients who fear food, I will test to rule out food allergies just to validate which foods are safe for the patient to eat. If a patient's symptoms seem to be an overlap of IBS and food allergy, it is worthwhile to test. If a patient is perseverating over food and eating and genuinely convinced that their symptoms derive from a food allergy, it is my opinion that it is worth testing for them. However, pure IBS is not a food allergy.

Delayed allergy to food, in which the response is delayed sometimes a week or more after ingestion, is tested by observing the prick test with a delayed reading or by patch testing. For more information about food allergy skin testing and patch testing (see Chapter 3).

What Other Tests May Be Used?

Other tests that may be performed, depending on the symptoms and any warning symptoms that are present, include labs to check liver, pancreas, and kidney function, stool studies to check for infection or malabsorption of fat, colonoscopy and upper endoscopy, abdominal X-ray or abdominal CT scan, lactose intolerance test, and breath test for bacterial overgrowth.

Treatment Approach for IBS-D (Irritable Bowel Syndrome-Diarrhea Predominant)

My usual approach to IBS-D is to start with a FODMAP diet and a better probiotic and then add on medical therapy. Many patients can be greatly helped with these two conservative measures. However, if the symptoms persist, I have found the following treatments to be effective for my patients.

Rifaximin (Xifaxan), when used for 10-14 days at a dose of 550 mg twice daily, is believed to decrease the bacterial overgrowth that may increase the risk of diarrhea. While uncommon, it can have side effects like allergy, drug interactions, nausea, increased liver tests, peripheral edema, dizziness, fatigue, and ascites; can increase the risk of bleeding; can cause bacterial diarrhea and colitis, headache, taste loss, weight decrease, myalgias; and should be used with care in the case of patients with liver failure and not at all during pregnancy or anticipated pregnancy or lactation. Rifaximin is only FDA-approved for adults with IBS but is approved for children 12 years and older with traveler's diarrhea.

Eluxadoline (Viberzi) is FDA-approved for treatment of adults with IBS-D as well. The typical adult dose is 100 mg twice daily, but this can be reduced to 75 mg twice daily in patients with severe kidney or liver impairment, intolerance of the higher dose, or who are receiving certain interfering medications. It is contraindicated in certain patients with biliary and gallbladder issues, patients with alcoholism or pancreatitis, or patients with severe constipation, as they may develop a bowel obstruction. Side effects include allergic reaction, constipation, pancreatitis, gallbladder spasm, nausea, vomiting, abdominal pain, upper respiratory tract infections, nasopharyngitis, flatulence, abdominal distension, impaired liver function, fatigue, rash, bronchitis, and dizziness. Viberzi is currently indicated for adults.

Metronidazole (Flagyl) can also be used to treat IBS-D and has been helpful for some patients, but is not technically FDA-approved for this purpose. The typical recommended dose is 400 mg three times daily for 10-14 days. Side effects include allergy, dizziness, headache, diarrhea, vomiting, nausea, abdominal pain, cramping, loss of appetite, constipation, headache, weight loss, dry mouth, changes in taste including metallic taste, fevers, mouth sores, pain with urination, brain disease and seizures, tingling/prickling sensations that may become permanent, unsteady gait, and mood changes. Kidney function should be monitored. Metronidazole has multiple serious drug interactions. Children under 12 years old should not be prescribed metronidazole.

Alosetron hydrochloride (Lotronex) is used to relax the colon and slow movement through the colon in adult women with IBS-D (not men). It has many drug interactions that need to be discussed ahead of time before deciding to use it. Side effects can be severe. They include but are not limited to allergy, ischemic colitis (decreased blood flow to the bowel), severe constipation, upset stomach, swollen stomach, and hemorrhoids. Using alosetron is considered only when other treatments fail. Alosetron is not currently used to treat children.

Medications for IBS-C (Irritable Bowel Syndrome-Constipation Predominant)

Linaclotide (Linzess) increases fluid secretion into the bowel to increase the fluid in the stool. It is only indicated for adults and children down to six years old with IBS-C. Side effects include allergy, diarrhea (although taking 30-60 minutes before eating can help), gas and bloating, abdominal pain, and abdominal distension.

Prucalopride (Motegrity) is a serotonin receptor agonist for adults with chronic idiopathic constipation and comes in 1 mg and 2 mg daily doses. Side effects include allergic reaction, rash, hives, facial swelling, intestinal perforation or obstruction, and severe inflammatory conditions of the intestinal tract such as Crohn's disease, ulcerative colitis, and toxic megacolon/megarectum. Prucalopride is not currently used in children.

Lubiprostone (Amitiza) is approved for women 18 years old and over with IBS-C and can help increase fluid in the stool. It is dosed at 8 mcg twice daily for IBS-C and 24 mcg twice daily for chronic idiopathic constipation. It needs to be reduced for patients with liver dysfunction. Side effects include allergic reaction, nausea, diarrhea, vomiting, shortness of breath, bowel obstruction, headache, abdominal pain and distention, flatulence, dry mouth, headache, swelling, and chest discomfort or pain. Lubiprostone is not currently used in children.

Reducing Stress and Getting Emotional Support Can Be Very Helpful

Another factor that affects IBS is stress. Reducing your child's stress and learning to avoid them "putting their stress" in their gut can help; cognitive behavioral therapy is an effective method for this type of learning.

Stress is a very real medical reality. It is not considered as often as it should be, perhaps due to our lack of recognition due to lack of training in the medical field. In my experience, stress is involved in many disease states and also increases the intensity of multiple disease processes. Stress is one of the root triggers of diseases such as migraine, hives, infections, and poor immune response.

Many would argue that stress is not the true cause of medical disease. I disagree. As an example, I walked into an appointment with a patient who was aware she was going to get the first shot of a drug for her illness that day. When I walked in, I did not have the drug with me, nor did I have any needles—I was just going in to chat with her and perform a quick exam. The minute she saw me—I had just opened the door—she passed out. I took her blood pressure, and it was excessively low. How did this happen? Stress. In medicine, we call this a vasovagal reaction.

The brain is a powerful, powerful instrument, one that has not been fully harnessed by modern medicine but really should be. Know that it is so important to keep your child's stress in check and also to remain positive.

Supplements That May Be Helpful for Gastrointestinal Upset and Pain

1. Peppermint oil manufactured as a food has been shown in several studies to help relieve the pain, constipation, bloating, and gas of IBS for some patients. There has not been much data for children under eight years old. Thus far, peppermint oil appears to be safe when used for up to eight weeks. It can cause an allergic reaction, dry mouth, nausea, vomiting, and reflux for rare patients. Caution: Most peppermint oils are not safe to ingest. Consult your child's physician for recommended sources.

   I will also note that peppermint oil as well as other "essential oils" should be used with caution. One of my patients consumed one too many pieces (a small handful) of homemade candy that contained peppermint oil and became extremely ill afterward, and required emergency room care. Please review all medications and medicinal use of all supplements, including essential oils, with your child's physician.

2. Tricyclic antidepressants may be helpful for those patients with diarrhea and abdominal pain and may be a bonus for those patients with depression. These drugs may regulate gut motility but have many side effects and drug interactions that should be reviewed before taking.

3. Selective Serotonin Reuptake Inhibitors (SSRIs) may also influence gut motility and can be helpful in a subset of patients with pain and constipation with or without depression.

4. For those patients who also have bile acid malabsorption, a bile acid binder like cholestyramine can help control diarrhea by binding bile acid, which can be irritating to the colon.

5. Anti-diarrhea medications, like loperamide, can be helpful for occasional diarrhea.
6. Fiber supplements with plenty of fluids can help with constipation.
7. Occasional laxatives can help with constipation.
8. Antispasmodics such as dicyclomine can decrease gut motility and help with diarrhea.

Lifestyle Modifications

Some of the recommended modifications that can be very helpful for IBS are:

1. Reduce stress. Stress is a common trigger for a flare of IBS.
2. Exercise regularly. This also helps reduce stress but can additionally normalize intestinal contractions.
3. Avoid gas-producing foods. Some foods promote gas and they should be avoided or reduced to a non-problematic level.
4. Eat regularly. Try not to skip meals or eat sporadically. This will help normalize intestinal function.
5. Once you know your child's triggers, avoid them.
6. Modify the fiber in your child's diet. Start low and slowly increase.
7. Drink plenty of water and keep your child hydrated.
8. Get regular sleep. This helps regulate bowel function and decrease stress.
9. Repleting zinc and vitamin D deficiencies, if found.
10. Consider adding a tailor-made probiotic.

IBS Can Be Helped

One of my poor patients, a teenage girl with IBS, noticed that every time she had cow's milk, she developed gas, bloating, distention, and loose stools. She would literally become sick from milk. All she had to do was cut down on the amount of milk and milk products she consumed and the symptoms disappeared. Some patients become so bloated they look nine months pregnant, but it is their intestine that is full of air. Can you imagine how much that hurts every time your child eats? That cannot make him/her enthusiastic to eat.

Many patients have to go through life knowing where bathrooms are ahead of time so they can time their eating and bathroom use. Many don't make it to the bathroom or may suddenly leave because they have stooled on themselves from diarrhea. The pain and embarrassment are unspeakable for some of these patients. When they are in the middle of a flare, they may have to skip some of life's most important events and interactions.

If your child has any of these symptoms, find an expert that can help.

Strategies to Help Pediatric Patients

As with adults, improving stress, diet, exercise, attempting a FODMAP diet, increasing fiber in the diet, and cognitive behavior therapy or other gut-directed therapies may be helpful as adjunct and conservative measures to manage intolerance.

Medication for Pediatric Patients

Hyoscyamine can be used in patients as young as two years of age to decrease gut motility and help with diarrhea. Side effects include allergy, palpitations, confusion and hallucination, dehydration and constipation, thirst, flushing, hot and dry skin, decreased sweating, headaches, sensitivity to light, palpitations, and difficulty with vision.

Loperamide reduces gut contractions and thereby increases the time for food to move through the gut, which can be very helpful to manage diarrhea in children two years old and older. Side effects include allergy, constipation, abdominal fullness and pain, palpitations, dizziness, and fainting.

Acid blockers may be helpful to manage abdominal pain in children. Some can be used in children as young as one month old. Side effects include allergic reaction, abdominal pain, nausea, vomiting, diarrhea, palpitations, headaches, constipation, and diarrhea. Famotidine can be used for patients beginning at six years of age and nizatidine can be used beginning at age 12.

Proton-pump inhibitors (PPIs), also used to decrease acid, can be helpful for abdominal pain. Some can be used for patients beginning at one month of age. Side effects include allergic reaction, abdominal pain, nausea, vomiting, diarrhea, fatigue, headache, dizziness, and rash. Some PPIs can be used to treat patients as young as one year old.

Antispasmodics such as dicyclomine can decrease gut motility and help with diarrhea. Dicyclomine can be used for patients who are six months old or older.

Linaclotide (Linzess) increases fluid secretion into the bowel, making it useful for IBS-C (see above). It is indicated for use by those six years old and older. Common side effects include diarrhea, stomach pain, gas, bloating, heartburn, vomiting, headache, and cold-like symptoms. Linaclotide can be used in patients that are two years old and older.

Antibiotics such as metronidazole and Rifaximin (Xifaxan) (see above) can help with bacterial overgrowth or bacteria-induced diarrhea. They are not specifically indicated for children with IBS but do have FDA indications for patients of 12 years of age and older for other reasons.

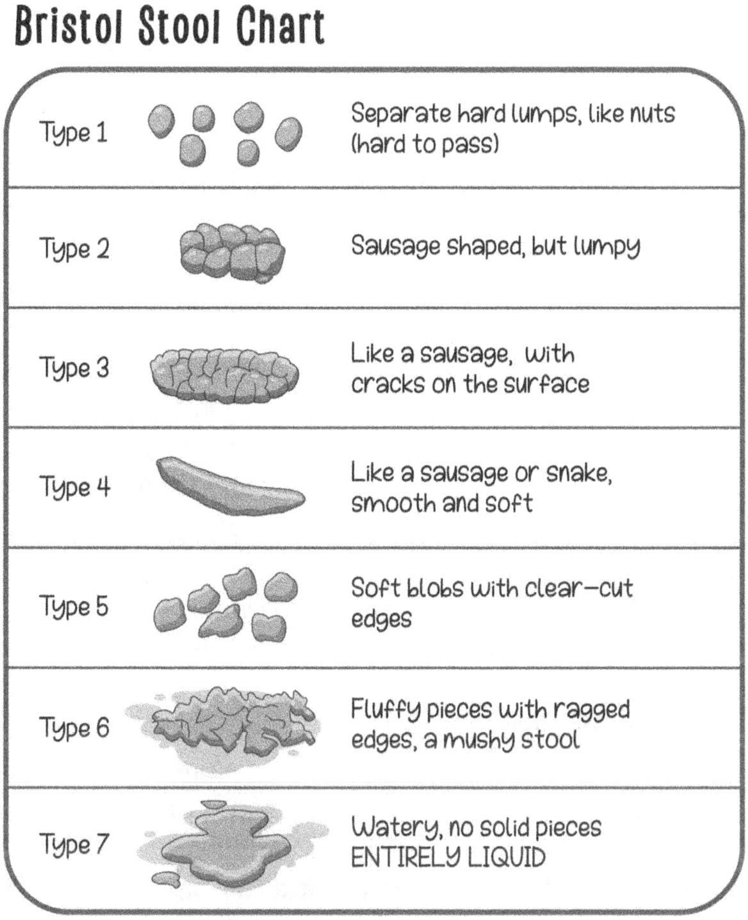

Bristol Stool Chart

Type 1		Separate hard lumps, like nuts (hard to pass)
Type 2		Sausage shaped, but lumpy
Type 3		Like a sausage, with cracks on the surface
Type 4		Like a sausage or snake, smooth and soft
Type 5		Soft blobs with clear-cut edges
Type 6		Fluffy pieces with ragged edges, a mushy stool
Type 7		Watery, no solid pieces ENTIRELY LIQUID

Figure 57: This chart shows the Bristol Stool Classifications. Type 1-2 is constipation; Type 3 is normal approaching constipation; Type-4 is normal; Type 5 is normal approaching diarrhea; and Type 6-7 is diarrhea.

Food Intolerance Symptoms May Also Result from Macronutrient Malabsorption

Carbohydrate malabsorption

Dysfunction of carbohydrate absorption is probably the most common type of macronutrient malabsorption. Symptoms like those of IBS include nausea, diarrhea and/or constipation, bloating, abdominal distention, and pain.

Besides the well-defined FODMAPs, other sugars consumed out of proportion to the patient's ability to break them down with digestive enzymes will result in the same symptoms. Aside from the six FODMAPs defined by Monash University, galactose, trehalose, and sucrose, when consumed out of proportion to galactosidase, trehalase, and sucrase, also allow the sugars to be delivered undigested to the intestine where the resident bacteria process them by fermentation, which creates gas and bloating. The undigested sugars create water fluxes that result in diarrhea. Trehalase is found in mushrooms, shellfish, honey, and yeast. Galactose is found in beets, chewing gum, avocado, dairy, and is produced by most microorganisms. Sucrose is found in fruits and vegetables.

Reasons for carbohydrate malabsorption syndrome

- Inflammation of the small intestine—from celiac disease, Crohn's disease, or ulcerative colitis—results in the same poor absorption of carbohydrates.
- Tropical sprue is an infection from bacteria (such as Klebsiella, E. coli, and Enterobacter) that tends to occur in tropical and subtropical climates and results in the same issues with malabsorption of carbohydrates as well as folate and B12.
- Similarly, infection with typical food-borne illnesses can cause inflammation of the intestine and result in malabsorption (see bacterial malabsorption, Chapter 20).
- When digestive enzymes are deficient or non-functional, carbohydrates cannot be broken down efficiently and are, therefore, not absorbed. Example: Pancreatic amylase breaks down starch and glycogen to their constituent simple sugars. This results in starch and glycogen intolerance.
- If a significant length of intestine is left after surgery, starch and glycogen intolerance can develop. Overgrowth of non-beneficial bacteria, such as in small intestinal bowel overgrowth (SIBO), will also cause starch and glycogen intolerance.
- Intestinal lymphangiectasia is a disorder of the lymphatic system, the vessels of which are responsible for circulating the cells of the immune system, helping drain tissues, and absorbing fat and fat-soluble nutrients. This condition also causes or contributes to carbohydrate and other malabsorption syndromes.

Protein malabsorption

Symptoms of protein malabsorption include fatigue, bloating, abdominal discomfort, nausea, vomiting, weight loss, muscle weakness, swelling of the hands and feet, rash, foul-smelling stools, immune system dysfunction, and slowed growth.

Digestion of protein begins in the stomach with proteases, the enzymes that break down proteins. Pancreatic and small intestinal proteases continue this process. The products of protein digestion are amino acids, the form that can be absorbed in the small intestine.

Reasons for protein malabsorption syndrome

- Causes of protein malabsorption are similar to those for carbohydrates. When there is inflammation of the intestine, lymphangiectasia, inflammatory bowel disease, or resection of a critical part of the intestine, protein absorption is inhibited.
- When the proteases are dysfunctional or decreased or if the pancreas cannot secrete sufficient bicarbonate, as in the case of cystic fibrosis or pancreatitis, protein malabsorption can occur.

Fat malabsorption

Fat malabsorption is characterized by fatty, greasy stool. Fat metabolism starts in the mouth, where an enzyme known as lingual lipase begins the digestive process. The stomach and pancreas contribute more lipolytic enzymes and most of the ingested fat is broken down and absorbed by the time it reaches the small intestine. Bile, which is synthesized in the liver and released into the intestine by the gallbladder, helps absorb more. Bile and fat are then reabsorbed in the small intestine where they are recycled for reuse.

Reasons for fat malabsorption syndrome

- Disruptions of the pancreas by pancreatic insufficiency—as with cystic fibrosis, pancreatic cancer, and pancreatitis—cause a decrease in the pancreatic lipase enzyme and bicarbonate production, which is required for fat digestion and absorption.
- Inflammation or surgery that removes the part of the intestine essential to fat absorption or disruption of the lymphatic system can also lead to fat malabsorption.
- Increased stomach acid from Zollinger-Ellison disease prevents activation of enzymes essential to digest fatty acids.
- Impairment of bile acid synthesis or reabsorption due to liver or gallbladder disease can also lead to fat malabsorption.
- Small intestinal bacterial overgrowth (SIBO) may cause fat malabsorption if the bacteria deactivate bile acids.
- Other nutrient malabsorption
- If the portion of the gastrointestinal tract where specific vitamins, nutrients, or minerals are absorbed is damaged or inflamed, it may result in a nutrient deficiency. Because vitamins A, D, E, and K, iron, calcium, magnesium, zinc, vitamin C, thiamine, riboflavin, pyridoxine, and folate are absorbed in the duodenum, damage or removal of this area can result in these deficiencies.

- Similarly, loss or damage of the jejunum (second part of the small intestine) can result in deficiencies of the following nutrients which it absorbs: iron, calcium, magnesium, zinc, vitamin C, thiamine, riboflavin, pyridoxine, and folate.
- Damage or removal of the ileum (the final part of the small intestine) may result in B12 deficiency, as the ileum is where B12 is absorbed.

Metabolic Disorders

Favism (Glucose-6-phosphate dehydrogenase deficiency) is a deficiency in the enzyme that is critical for red blood cell function and in preventing oxidative damage to them. Patients with this hereditary deficiency cannot tolerate certain drugs and, on ingestion of fava beans or those drugs, can develop severe acute hemolytic anemia with accompanying jaundice, pallor, shortness of breath, abdominal pain, fever, chills, nausea, and, rarely, kidney failure. These symptoms occur within hours of ingestion of fava beans. The absence of the protective enzyme caused by this disorder is responsible for the damage and destruction of red cells.

There are other causes of metabolic issues, most of which are very rare and can be very serious or even life-threatening (*For more information, go to Medline Plus, National Library of Medicine,* https://medlineplus.gov/metabolicdisorders.html).

Inborn Errors of Metabolism

Inborn errors of metabolism (IEM) can be easily overlooked unless they are found during newborn screening. Not all IEMs are tested at newborn screening and not all states have the same newborn screening tests. IEMs frequently mimic other complex disease processes, presenting with a diverse group of symptoms involving multiple body systems at the same time, including neurological and gastrointestinal systems. This complexity makes diagnosis a challenge and prolongs the time to diagnosis; this is why IEMs are often a diagnosis of exclusion.

Many children with IEMs have difficulty processing various food components, the most common of which is lactase deficiency. However, in the case of IEMs, symptoms of food intolerance do not mean the child has food allergies or food toxicity. While lactase deficiency is not life-threatening, some IEMs are. These should be addressed with a specialist physician.

Reasons to Consider Inborn Errors of Metabolism as a Cause of Food Intolerance

All of the following symptoms and issues—especially when diagnosed at birth or at a young age or which result in a death of undetermined cause—are compatible with an IEM (Agana 2018):

- Seems to mimic recurrent sepsis, anoxic encephalopathy, and/or apparent brain damage from low oxygen or from toxic ingestion.
- Presents like a food intolerance, food aversion, food allergy, or food toxicity.
- Continues, despite treatment for the suspected disease process.
- Laboratory tests cannot confirm the suspected disease process.
- Patterns include acute, chronic, recurrent, or progressive.
- Can occur even with a negative family and/or genetic history of metabolic disorders.

Bacterial Malabsorption

Chronic diarrhea, which may or may not result in severe illness or weight loss, is the most common symptom of bacterial malabsorption. Giardia lamblia is the most common cause and results from consuming contaminated food or water. The most common causes of food-borne illness in the United States are norovirus, salmonella, clostridium perfringens, campylobacter, hepatitis A, staphylococcus aureus, listeria, E. coli, and vibrio cholera (CDC 2020).

While traveling, the most common causes of food- and water-borne illness are E. coli, campylobacter jejuni, shigella, salmonella, aeromonas, plesiomonas, arcobacter, laribacter, bacteroides fragilis, norovirus, rotavirus, astrovirus, giardiasis, entamoeba histolytica, cyclospora, and dientamoeba fragilis (CDC 2021). Microsporidiosis is contracted by ingestion, inhalation, and direct contact with animals infected with this fungus. Cryptosporidium is caused by consuming contaminated water, including that in swimming pools. Whipple's disease is caused by a bacterium that is consumed with contaminated food and is potentially a severe issue for immune-compromised patients.

Have you ever been to a foreign country and developed travelers' diarrhea shortly thereafter? I have, and it is a miserable way to end a vacation! Two of the most common causes of travelers' diarrhea are norovirus and giardiasis. Norovirus is famous (in a bad way) for causing diarrhea in people traveling on cruise ships. Giardiasis is commonly contracted when people drink water from wells and untreated water in other countries and untreated river water when camping. Just after we adopted my puppy, Huxley, he was diagnosed with giardial diarrhea, and this was not at all fun in a potty-training pup. While this is meant to be a fun comment, it also brings up the fact that some infection transmission can occur between a sick pet and his/her family. Asking about sick pets is one of the many inquiries I make when patients have gastrointestinal issues.

Probiotics Help Manage Causes of IBS and Other Intestinal Symptoms

We are in the infancy of understanding our microbiome, the bacterial population of the gut. However, what is becoming clear is that there is a good deal of "cross talk" between our gut and the good and bad gut bacteria that live there.

Certain types of bacteria are being implicated as causing certain disease states, including autism, allergy, atopic dermatitis, asthma, obesity, inflammatory bowel syndrome, etc.

In contrast, probiotics have been shown to be helpful in addressing causes of diarrhea, constipation, diverticula disease, irritable bowel syndrome, colic, and even some dental disorders. Further, probiotics have proven valuable in preventing necrotizing enterocolitis (a very serious form of bowel inflammation in infants) as well as antibiotic-associated diarrhea in hospitalized patients (Zhang 2022).

Some manufacturers produce customized "designer probiotics" by first assessing a patient's health needs and characterizing bacteria in their microbiome through stool studies before composing the final probiotic with their strains. The goal tends to be increasing the "good bacteria" at the expense of the bad and creating a varied microbiome that can be protective.

Caution before taking probiotics is advised for those patients who are immunocompromised, as some probiotics have harmful substances and bacteria other than what is listed on the label, so using a reputable vendor is highly recommended.

Warning Symptoms

Emergency symptoms include bloody or black stools, coughing up black blood, unintentional weight loss, early satiety, swallowing issues, sudden worsening of symptoms, onset after 50 years old, a family history of celiac disease, inflammatory bowel disease, or colon cancer.

Part 6: Toxic Effects of Food

Chapter 21

Toxic Effects of Foods: Eat What You Kill or Does What You Eat Kill You?

Chapter Preview

- What are some of the toxins found naturally in foods?
- Which toxins are created from cooking and food processing?
- What are some of the diseases that can be caused by toxins in foods?
- Which foods should we avoid to stay away from natural and introduced toxins?
- Food and drug interactions that can have toxic effects.

Food is rarely thought of as dangerous or life-threatening. However, toxins are naturally present in many foods and are more common than most people appreciate. For example, when food molds, mycotoxins are created that can cause illness and disease. Examples of the mycotoxins found in various foods are in the table below.

Toxic Substances That Naturally Occur in Food

We depend on food for survival. We take for granted that our food is safe, but a lot can happen between the time it is planted and the time it lands on our plate for dinner. Most of us have not experienced toxicity from food, short of perhaps an episode of food poisoning. However, even this can be frightening.

The chart below highlights the major fungal producers, hosts, toxic effects of mycotoxins, and maximum permitted levels in food as determined by the United States Food and Drug Administration (US FDA) and the European Union (EU).

Table 12

Toxic Effects of Certain Foods	
Food	**Toxic Effects**
Apple	Pulmonary congestion, edema, convulsions, dyspnea, gastrointestinal toxicity
Cereal-derived products, spices, wine	Nephrotoxic, carcinogenic, teratogenic, immunotoxic
Corn	Hepatotoxicity, cancer, pulmonary edema, leukoencephalomalacia
Corn, barley, wheat, rice	Infertility, abortion
Corn, nuts, cottonseed, peanuts	Hepatoxicity, immunosuppression, liver cancer
Corn, wheat, barley	Gastrointestinal toxicity, inflammation of the central nervous system
Milk, milk products	Hepatotoxicity, liver cancer, immunosuppression

Adapted from the following resources:
He T, Zhu J, Nie Y, Hu R, Wang T, Li P, Zhang Q, Yang Y. Nanobody technology for mycotoxin detection in the field of food safety: current status and prospects. *Toxins* (Basel). 2018;10(5):180. doi: 10.3390/toxins10050180. PMID: 29710823; PMCID: PMC5983236.

Mycotoxins	Major Producers	Maximum Level US FDA (mcg/kg)	Maximum Level EU (mcg/kg)
Patulin	P. expansus	50	10-50
Ochratoxin A (OTA)	Penicillium verrucosum, A. ochraceus	--	2-80
Fumonisins B1, B2, B3	Fusarium verticillioides, F. proliferatum	2000-4000	200-4000
Zearalenone	F. culmoraum, F. graninearum	--	20-400
Aflatoxins B1, B2, G1, G2	Aspergillus flavus, Aspergillus parasiticus	20	2-12 of B1, 4-15 of B2, G1, G2
Deoxynivalenol	F. graminearum, F. culmorum	1000	200-1750
Aflatoxin M1	Aspergillus parasiticus	0.5	

U.S. Food and Drug Administration. Mycotoxins: toxins found in food infected by certain molds or fungi. U.S. FDA website. Updated July 21, 2022. Accessed December 13, 2022. https://www.fda.gov/food/natural-toxins-food/mycotoxins.
European Food Safety Authority. Mycotoxins. European Food Safety Authority website. Updated 2020. Accessed December 13, 2022. https://www.efsa.europa.eu/en/topics/topic/mycotoxins.

Table 13

Natural Toxins Found in Foods and Their Effects

Food	Toxic Effects
Apricots, apples, peaches, almonds, lima beans, sorghum, bamboo roots	Nausea, vomiting, diarrhea, abdominal pain, cyanosis, hypotension, respiratory decompensation, dizziness, headache, seizure, coma, and death
Barracuda, king mackerel, black grouper, dog snapper	Nausea, vomiting, and neurologic symptoms
Cereals, grains, honey, eggs, coffee, cacao seeds, tea leaves, tomatoes, potatoes	Cancer
Cinnamon (but not Ceylon)	Severe rash when exposed to light, gastrointestinal side effects, liver damage, and cancer
Citrus plants, celery, and parsnips	Severe rash when exposed to light, gastrointestinal side effects, liver damage, and cancer
Fruits and vegetables, meats, fish, shellfish, dried mushrooms	Nausea, vomiting, diarrhea, abdominal pain, pain and burning of the esophagus, shortness of breath, fatigue, myeloid cancer, cancer of sinuses and nasopharynx
Honey, home canning, opened cans that have lost their seal	18-24 hours after consumption, constipation, floppy movements, muscle weakness, difficulty moving head
Kidney beans, other beans	Severe stomach ache, vomiting, diarrhea
Mushrooms	Blurred vision, increased salivation, vomiting, diarrhea, abdominal pain, confusion and hallucinations, liver and kidney damage, death
Mussels, scallops, oysters	Diarrhea, vomiting, paresthesia, paralysis, death
Tomatoes, potatoes, eggplants, plants of the nightshade family	Nausea, vomiting, diarrhea, abdominal pain and cramping, dizziness and headache, heart rhythm disturbances, burning throat, eczema, thyroid issues, death
Shark, barramundi, swordfish, bluefin tuna, orange roughy, tilefish, and king mackerel	Neurologic effects; difficulty hearing and seeing, hallucinations, difficulty moving and speaking, emotional lability, immune dysfunction, liver and kidney disease
Teas, coffee	Diarrhea, insomnia, headache, gastrointestinal complaints
Tuna, mackerel, marlin, bonita, skipjack	Anaphylaxis-like: nausea, vomiting, diarrhea, flushing, hypotension, headache, shortness of breath, wheezing, chest tightness, swelling of throat or tongue
Wine, yogurt, fruit juice, pureed fruit, baby food, preserved vegetables, soy sauce, vinegar, anything fermented with yeast	"Hangover"; rapid heartrate, headache, upset stomach, memory impairment, irreversible DNA damage, breast, liver and oral cancer

Adapted from the following resources:
World Health Organization. Natural toxins in food. World Health Organization website. Updated May 9, 2018. Accessed December 13, 2022. https://www.who.int/news-room/fact-sheets/detail/natural-toxins-in-food.

Toxin	Producer	Comments
Cyanogenic glycosides	>2000 plant species	Specific plants listed are especially important
Ciguatoxin	Dinoflagellates	Known as ciguatera fish poisoning
Pyrrolizidine alkaloids	Boraginaceae, Asteraceae, Fabaceae	Risk has not been fully evaluated
Coumarins	Cinnamon (but not Ceylon)	Mostly after skin exposure, systemic effects can occur when high quantities consumed
Furocoumarins	Citrus plants, celery, and parsnips	Mostly after skin exposure, systemic effects can occur when large quantities consumed
Formaldehyde	Yeast	
Botulinum spores	Clostridia botulinum	Can progress to death
Lectins	Kidney beans, other beans	Destroyed when soaked and boiled thoroughly
Muscimol and muscarine	Mushrooms	Cooking or peeling does not inactivate; avoid wild mushrooms
Algal toxins, microcystin	Algae, during bloom	No smell or taste; not destroyed by heating or freezing
Glycoalkaloids (solanine and chaconine)	Produced in the green and bitter-tasting parts, like the buds of potatoes	Produced under stress, bruising, UV light and on attack from pests and infection
Mercury	Accumulates in tissues of fish; large predatory fish also consume when they eat smaller fish	
Caffeine	Teas, coffee	
Histamine	Bacteria on scombroid fish convert histidine to histamine	Fresh, canned, or frozen
Acetaldehyde	Yeast	

U.S. Food and Drug Administration. Natural toxins in food. U.S. FDA website. Updated July 22, 2022. Accessed December, 13, 2022. https://www.fda.gov/food/chemical-contaminants-metals-pesticides-food/natural-toxins-food.

We live in an age of convenience. We have reduced our search for food from every time we need to eat to once a day, and from that to purchasing it at the grocery store once per week. To maintain this level of convenience, food is processed in order to be fit for our consumption for longer periods, to prevent food poisoning, and to avoid other adverse health effects. The net effect is that we have traded one set of problems for another due to the way we source and prepare our food for the sake of convenience.

◆ ◆ ◆

There are so many ways food can be dangerous.

When my brother was just six months old and newly started on baby food, my mother brought home baby food for him, which he intensely enjoyed as this was more satisfying for him than formula or milk. One day, my mother served him baby food out of a jar. She did not hear the typical "pop" from the container but did not think anything of it. Within a day, my brother became ill and "floppy." He developed muscle weakness and lost control of his head and movements. My mother instantly brought him to the emergency room. He was diagnosed with salmonella poisoning and treated with antibiotics. Salmonella is not only dangerous because it is a nasty bacteria and wreaks havoc on a patient's gut, it also produces multiple toxins that remain viable long after this bacteria is gone.

When the emergency department physician noted that one of the most common sources of food poisoning is improperly canned food, my mother realized the culprit was the jar of baby food that did not pop when she opened it.

Since then, whenever she spotted people at the grocery store opening jars and tasting the contents, they would endure her lecture on the consequences of giving someone food poisoning. She will also give the opened jar to the store manager so it cannot be used. Although I do not personally recall this incident, I know it was traumatic because my mother repeated the story many times while we were growing up and I have personally witnessed one of her lectures to unsuspecting food tasters at the grocery store.

As the World Health Organization describes, there are many natural toxins. These are produced by plants, algae, and plankton as their normal defense against predation, as natural pesticides, or under conditions of stress.

◆ ◆ ◆

Table 14

Health Effects of Food Processing

Processing method	Reason	Effect
Addition of nitrates and nitrites	As preservatives	Allergic reactions, migraines
Addition of benzoates	As preservatives	Allergic reactions
Butylated hydroxytoluene (BHT), Butylated hydroxyanisole (BHA)	As preservatives	Contact dermatitis, hives
Bisphenol A (BPA)	Present in plastic food and drink containers	Implicated in infertility, diabetes, obesity, immune system dysfunction
Artificial trans fat	Unsaturated oils made into solid fat (such as margarine)	Cardiotoxic effects, inflammation
Heating of highly refined vegetable oils causes aldehyde reduction	Cooking	Cancer causing; because they contain high amounts of omega-3, if consumed out of proportion to omega-6 are also proinflammatory
Production of polycyclic aromatic hydrocarbons	Burning and smoking meat	Toxic, cancer-causing
Addition of monosodium glutamate	As a preservative	"Chinese Restaurant Syndrome": headache, chest tightness, nausea, diarrhea, flushing of the neck, profuse sweating, asthma attack
Addition of sulfites	As a preservative	May provoke asthma attacks, anaphylaxis, and migraines in various sensitive patients
Addition of methylparaben, ethylparaben, propylparaben, and butylparaben	As preservatives	May cause contact dermatitis
Addition of tartrazine	As a yellow dye	May cause anaphylaxis, asthma, hives, swelling and other allergic reactions
Addition of carmine (extracted from Coccus cacti bug)	As a red dye	May cause anaphylaxis, asthma, hives, swelling and other allergic reactions
Addition of sugar	As an additive to sweeten food	Triggers insulin resistance and increases risk of obesity and inflammation, increases dopamine in the brain, making it addictive

Adapted from: U.S. Food and Drug Administration. Process contaminants in foods. U.S. FDA website. Updated February 25, 2022. Accessed December 13, 2022. https://www.fda.gov/food/chemical-contaminants-food/process-contaminants-food

Table 15

Food and Drug Interactions	
Food	**Drug**
Alcohol	Many
Alcohol	Nonsteroidal anti-inflammatories and Acetaminophen
Alcohol products	Acetaminophen
Black licorice	Glycyrrhizic acid and glycyrrhetic acid
Caffeine	Multiple drugs
Charbroiled food	Warfarin
Cooked onions	Warfarin
Cow's milk	Various drugs
Cranberry juice	Many (anything metabolized through specific liver enzymes)
Diet high in carbohydrates	Multiple
Diet high in polyunsaturated fatty acids	Multiple
Excess iron	Multiple
Fat, fatty meal	Vitamin A, D, E, K, multiple others
Foods with tyramine (aged meats and cheeses)	Monoamine oxidases
Grapefruit	Many (anything metabolized through specific liver enzymes)
Green leafy vegetables	Vitamin K
Herbal supplements	Multiple drugs
High protein diet	Many
High-protein diet	Multiple
Milk and dairy	Calcium ions, magnesium ions

Nature of interaction	Effect
Alters absorption, depending on solubility	Alters absorption
Increases levels of drug	Increases risk of liver damage, failure, and bleeding
Increases acetaminophen levels	Hepatotoxicity, liver failure, death
Increases cortisol	Increased sodium, decreased potassium, hypertension, swelling, other steroid effects
Affects absorption, distribution, and elimination	Increases risk of drug toxicity
Decreases warfarin activity	Decreases efficacy of drugs
Increases warfarin activity	Can cause bleeding
Reduces bioavailability	Decreases effective levels
Inhibits function of specific liver enzymes	Decreases detoxification of these drugs by the liver
Inhibits specific liver enzymes	Alters metabolism
Increases specific liver enzymes	Increases degradation of effected drugs
Various effects on specific liver enzymes	Alters metabolism; excess may cause damage to entire system
Increases absorption of these fat-soluble vitamins; increases bioavailability of some drugs and decreases bioavailability of others; decreases serum concentration of other drugs, decreases activity of liver; increases specific liver enzymes	Elevates serum levels of vitamins, may lead to toxicity, increases or decreases availability or serum levels, prevents degradation; excess can increase activity of mixed function oxidase system and therefore metabolism; deficiency can decrease MFO system
Tyramine not digested, releases neurotransmitters from synapses that result in uncontrolled blood pressure	Hypertensive crisis
Inhibits function of specific liver enzymes	Decreases detoxification of these drugs by the liver; increases bioavailability
Interferes with warfarin metabolism	Lowers INR; may develop thromboembolic complications
May have same or contradictory effect, alters absorption, distribution, bioavailability, and elimination	Variable effects including synergism or counteracting
Increases albumin, which binds to many drugs	Usually decreases bioavailability
Raises albumin and can decrease bioavailability of some drugs; can alter enzyme induction	Changes bioavailability and therefore efficacy of some drugs; can alter rate of metabolism (excess can increase and deficiency can decrease rate of metabolism)
Prevents antibiotic absorption	Interferes with efficacy of antibiotic

Table 16

Food and Drug Interactions	
Food	**Drug**
Orange juice	Multiple
Pectin (fruits, especially pears, apples, guavas, quince, plums, gooseberries, oranges, and other citrus fruits)	Acetaminophen
Riboflavin	Multiple
Sesame seeds	Tamoxifen and others
Thiamine	Multiple
Vitamin C	Multiple
Vitamin E	Multiple

Bushra R, Aslam N, Khan AY. Food-drug interactions. *Oman Med J.* 2011; 26(2):77-83. doi: 10.5001/omj.2011.21. PMID: 22043389; PMCID: PMC3191675.

Can Food Cause Cancer?

One in every two men and one in every three women in the United States will develop cancer at some point in their lifetime (ACS 2010).

As an allergist-immunologist with prior training and experience in internal medicine, I was aware that food can be a potential source of carcinogens. However, until I did research for this book, I assumed that if I took reasonable steps to eat "clean," I—and more importantly, my family—would be fine. Even the possibility that food may cause cancer was frightening and surprising to learn. While most of this book contains information drawn from my training and experience, this topic is mostly new to me. This research I provide is all published by governmental agencies—please do your due diligence by reading my sources if you do not believe me.

The most disappointing and shocking aspect of food toxicity to me is that our most brilliant and creative minds have made such incredible strides for us in food science, which is wonderful. However, we do not "test before we treat." We seem to just assume the medication, chemical, or food is safe to use until many years later, when the substance, product, byproduct, or chemical becomes associated with cancer, or autism, or neurologic issues, or some other terrible condition. This surprises me because I am in the medical field, which is heavily regulated.

I would never think to use a drug on a human without understanding the purpose behind the creation of the drug, the way it works in the body, its side effects, and the risks and rewards of using it. I study each drug and share that information with

Nature of interaction	Effect
Acidity decreases intestinal absorption	Decreases absorption of multiple drugs
Delays absorption and onset	Decreases absorption and time to work
In excess, decreases specific liver enzymes	Alters metabolism
Interferes with and delays absorption	Decreases efficacy
Excess decreases, deficiency increases activity of specific liver enzymes	Alters metabolism
Affects multiple specific liver enzymes	Alters metabolism
Deficiency decreases specific liver enzymes	Decreases metabolism

the patient so they can make an informed decision. At the same time, we are all innocently eating food and drinking beverages without understanding their short and long-term health implications. It is a bit horrifying to me.

I am especially concerned because a number of my family members have been diagnosed with autism; I know this is becoming more and more common. I see many more patients with autism than ever before. While I understand there is some genetic component to autism, could the rate of autism be increased by something in our diet? This is, pardon the pun, food for thought.

The number of patients and families that come to me for help with IBS and food intolerance has skyrocketed in the last five years as well. Why? I am not entirely sure, but my theory is that we, as a society, have created some exposure—unintentionally, I am sure—that has altered our gut in some way and has contributed to these problems. My best guess is that this change is predominantly, but maybe not solely, in the microbiome.

The U.S. and the E.U. Monitor Carcinogen Levels in Food

Two intergovernmental agencies—the National Toxicology Program of the Department of Health and Human Services (HHS) and the International Agency for Research on Cancer (IARC) of the World Health Organization (WHO)—conduct and coordinate research into the causes of cancer. They also collect and publish surveillance data regarding the occurrence of cancer worldwide.

Annually, the HHS publishes the National Toxicology Program's (NTP) report on carcinogens, which contains the results of their ongoing research of chemical, physical, and biological agents, mixtures, and exposure circumstances that are known or reasonably anticipated to cause cancer in humans. It then labels them as either *known human carcinogens* or *reasonably anticipated to be a human carcinogen*, as follows:

- **Known human carcinogens** - This label indicates that there is sufficient evidence of carcinogenicity from studies in humans to indicate a causal relationship between exposure to the agent, substance, or mixture and human cancer (NTP 2011).
- **Reasonably anticipated to be a human carcinogen** - This label indicates that a causal interpretation is credible, but:
  - Alternative explanations and confounding factors cannot be excluded or the carcinogenicity data is from animal experiments;
  - There is less than sufficient evidence of carcinogenicity in humans or animals but the agent is structurally related to a human carcinogen;
  - The substance is reasonably anticipated to be a human carcinogen; or
  - There is enough information to indicate that it acts through a mechanism that would cause cancer in humans (NTP 2011).

In the appendix at the end of this book is a six-page summary of potentially carcinogenic agents that can currently be found in foods, those foods with the highest concentration of the agents, and their potential side effects. Many agents, such as benzidine in food dyes, have been found and banned because they were listed by the NTP or IARC. As those substances are no longer permitted in foods, they are no longer on the list. However, they were potentially in our food supply for a long time. As hard as the scientists at the NTP and IARC work, it is a long process to develop enough scientific evidence to prove that something should be labeled as a carcinogen. If I were the owner of a business that made food that was under consideration as a carcinogen, I would be grateful for this careful process. However, is this the way we should review our food? Perhaps proving that it is safe for general consumption should come first. More food for thought.

Chapter 22

Food Aversion:
You Aren't What You Don't Eat

Aversion to food may occur if the patient becomes ill shortly after consuming a uniquely-flavored food. Thus, the taste of the food is associated with symptoms of an illness. This is also known as conditioned taste aversion. Representation of the food may produce symptoms such as nausea or reproduce the original symptoms and cause the patient to avoid those foods.

This is a genuine medical condition and should not be dismissed.

Conditioned taste aversion (or learned avoidance) is believed to be an adaptive trait to protect your child from eating foods that may contain toxins or bacteria that could cause illness and potentially death. As well, food deprivation during a period of bacterial infection may increase survival and decrease mortality (Chambers 2018).

Examples include:

- Inability to eat during cancer therapies.
- It is believed that high estrogen states may promote a similar restriction of food, such as anorexia nervosa (Chambers 2018).
- Timing is important. The closer in time food consumption occurs with an adverse event, even if unrelated, the more likely it is to be implicated as a cause of the event and the more likely it is to cause an aversion.
- In cases of infection, the cause may be hormones of inflammation known as cytokines.
- For some toxic substances like chemotherapy, the trigger may also be hormonal (Chambers 2018).

◆ ◆ ◆

I developed a food aversion myself when I was about 14 years old. Being very curious about the rice cakes that my mother brought home and wanting something quick to eat one morning before school, I slathered a few rice cakes with peanut butter and ate them quickly before school. By second period, my abdomen was in extreme pain, and I developed nausea, vomiting, and a fever quickly thereafter. My high school sent me home. My mom let me sleep, but I was worse the next morning. She poked my belly, noticed the pain localizing in the right lower quadrant, and called my doctor. I was sent to the hospital for an emergency appendectomy that afternoon. It took me 35 years to try another rice cake and I probably will never love them. This is a prime example of how an aversion develops: a very negative experience becomes associated with a food and creates an extreme distaste.

◆ ◆ ◆

Recommendations for navigating food aversion

Many children with autism will have many food aversions, likely due to their heightened sensory sensitivities. It may be the taste, texture, or smell that overstimulates them, but it is truly unpleasant and should not be discounted, nor should liking something that they have an aversion to be forced. It can, however, be navigated carefully.

There are many recommendations I have for parents of children with sensory issues that result in a restricted diet:

1. Understand the sensory issues. It may be a sound you take for granted (a Styrofoam container opening), or the overstimulation caused by loud noises, bright lights, and/or many children running around in a gymnasium during lunch, or a texture, or even the color.
2. Make the dinner experience as minimally stimulating as possible:
   i. Avoid bright lights.
   ii. Avoid loud noises.
   iii. Don't let the other kids run around during dinner.
   iv. Except on special occasions, reserve dinner time just for family.
3. Find a way to get your child invested in what they eat: have them prepare it with you.
4. Make preparing and eating food fun:
   i. Consider making a miniature scene, with broccoli trees and carrot stick houses, or a face with a red pepper smile and sliced olive eyes and a grape tomato nose, or shape animals out of tomatoes and grapes and olives.
   ii. Think about making kabobs.

    iii. Use cookie cutters.

5. Take the child shopping. Point out something with a crazy name (moon drop grapes, dragon fruit) or something new every time. Have your child pick one item they want to try.

6. Ask your child why they do not like something. It may give you insight into sensitivities that will be particularly tough to overcome right away.

7. Get your child's opinion.

8. Have your child invent new recipes or name recipes.

9. Do not force the issue, but gently push.

10. Do not worry about what your child eats or if it does not make sense to you. If they eat salad without salad dressing, for example, it is healthier and does not matter that you would not do this.

11. Consider allowing use of a moderate amount of low-salt soy sauce, barbecue sauce, and ketchup.

Part 7: Diseases Associated with Food

Which Came First: The Chicken or the Egg Allergy?

How Foods Impact Select Diseases

Twenty percent of patients alter their diets to reduce allergic reactions, but many reactions are adverse responses or side effects rather than food allergy (Sicherer 2010). There are clear adverse symptoms in both cases, but those from food allergy are the direct result of an immune response to the food. For some reason, some patients are upset when I tell them they are not allergic and that they had an adverse reaction. This does not make the adverse response less real or invalidate what is going on. It also is not an indication that the adverse reaction is not a genuine medical problem.

Chapter 23

Food for Thought:
Food Allergy and Autism

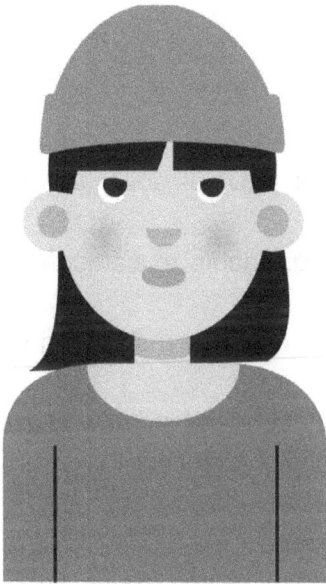

It is estimated that 84.1% of children with autism studied had some gastrointestinal issue compared with 31.2% neurotypical controls (Horvath 2002). Food allergy increases general irritability and results in poorer functional outcomes in those who have autism spectrum disorder (ASD). The association between food allergy and ASD was significant in all subgroups, including age, sex, and race/ethnicity (Xu 2018). Most strikingly, food allergy occurred in 11.25% of autists v. 4.25% of controls (Xu 2018). The CHARGE study (Childhood Autism Risks from Genetics and Environment) also suggested that food allergies and sensitivities were more common in autistic children, especially those with higher scores consistent with the Autism Aberrant Behavior Checklist (Lyall 2015).

My own theory is the increased sensitivity to stimuli seen in ASD may cause autistic people to avoid certain foods and, furthermore, prolonged abstinence from those foods may result in increased sensitivity and increased likelihood of allergy. As well, it is my observation that increased food intolerance exists in our culture in general and the accompanying distention, loose stools/diarrhea, constipation, abdominal pain, and nausea is particularly uncomfortable and irritating to autistic children. Any perceived issue, whether severe from allergy or discomfort from intolerance, is felt profoundly by the hypersensitive autistic child, making them more likely to be aggravated from the stimulus. Autistic individuals also have a greater sensitivity to stimulus of any type and that includes the taste or texture of a food. For more advice on overcoming childhood food aversion, especially in an autistic individual, see Chapter 22.

Important Things to Know about a Person with Autism

Social communication and interaction

A child or adult with autism spectrum disorder may have problems with social interaction and communication skills, and may exhibit any of these signs (CDC 2022):

- Fails to respond to their name or appears not to hear you at times
- Resists cuddling and holding, and seems to prefer playing alone, retreating into his or her own world
- Has poor eye contact and lacks facial expression
- Doesn't speak or has delayed speech, or loses previous ability to say words or sentences
- Can't start a conversation or keep one going; unable to participate in the "back and forth" way of conversing
- Speaks with an abnormal tone or rhythm and may use a singsong voice or robot-like speech
- Repeats words or phrases verbatim, but doesn't understand how to use them
- Doesn't appear to understand simple questions or directions
- Doesn't express emotions or feelings and appears unaware of others' feelings
- Doesn't point at or bring objects to share interest
- Inappropriately approaches a social interaction by being passive, aggressive, or disruptive
- Fixated on his/her specific interests and uninterested in others' interests
- Has difficulty recognizing nonverbal cues, such as interpreting other people's facial expressions, body postures or tone of voice

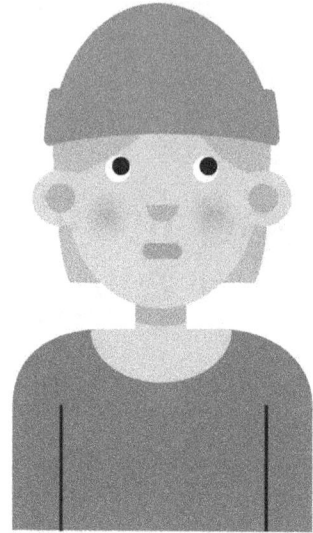

Patterns of behavior

A child or adult with autism spectrum disorder may have limited, repetitive patterns of behavior, interests or activities. Signs of this include:

- Repetitive movements (rocking, spinning, hand clapping)
- Performs activities that could cause self-harm (biting or head-banging)
- Disturbed at slightest change in routine
- Problem with coordination (movement patterns, such as clumsiness or walking on toes, and has odd, stiff or exaggerated body language)

- Fascinated by details of objects (spinning wheels of a toy car, doesn't understand the overall purpose or function of the object)
- Is unusually sensitive to light, sound or touch, may be indifferent to pain or temperature
- Doesn't engage in imitative or make-believe play
- Abnormal intensity or focus on objects
- Specific food preferences (eating only a few foods, or refusing foods with a certain texture

While this is a laundry list of "typical" symptoms, this condition is a spectrum and all people on the autism spectrum manifest the condition in different and unique ways.

What We've Learned about the Role of the Microbiome in Diseases

The microbiome, or the milieu of bacteria that make their home in our gut (as well as in our sinuses, lungs, and other areas of the body that communicate with the outside world) has been shown to be increasingly important in many disease states. While our understanding of the microbiome is still in its infancy, there are identifiable patterns that tend to characterize both disease states and states of wellness, the microbiome communicates with us and affects us, and the microbiome in one area communicates with the microbiomes in other areas of the body.

The microbiome has been most successfully studied and used to help control inflammatory bowel disease and help manage and sometimes solve irritable bowel disease and bacteria-associated diarrhea. Study of the microbiome in autism is relatively new but nonetheless important. For example, it has been shown that by using amino acids, the firmicutes to bacteroidetes ratio could be decreased in the small intestine, thus decreasing or modulating inflammation in the autistic person (van Sandelhof 2019).

A diet higher in branched-chain amino acids such as leucine, valine, and isoleucine decreased the higher proteobacteria levels in people with ASD as well as those patients with inflammatory colitis and inflammatory bowel disease (Sandelhof 2019). While a neuroprotective and anti-inflammatory diet reduces behavioral deficits in mice, it has not yet been completely validated in humans.

Foods and nutrients emphasized in this diet include:

- **Lysine** - Present in generous amounts in meat, egg, soy, black beans, quinoa, and pumpkin seeds.
- **Histidine** - Meat, fish, poultry, nuts, seeds, and whole grains contain large amounts of this nutrient.
- **High threonine** - foods include lean beef, pork, tuna, tofu, beans, milk, cheese, green peas, eggs, seeds, and nuts.

It is particularly disheartening to learn that food can be neurotoxic and may lead or contribute to autism and other neurodevelopmental issues. N-nitroso compounds, such as N-ethyl-N-nitrosourea (ENU), have been implicated in neurodevelopmental dysregulation as well as in neurocarcinogenesis, increasing the risk of gliomas (Bulnes 2021). ENU is used in flavorings, colorings, and preservatives.

Chapter 24

Red is Not My Favorite Color: Foods and Rosacea

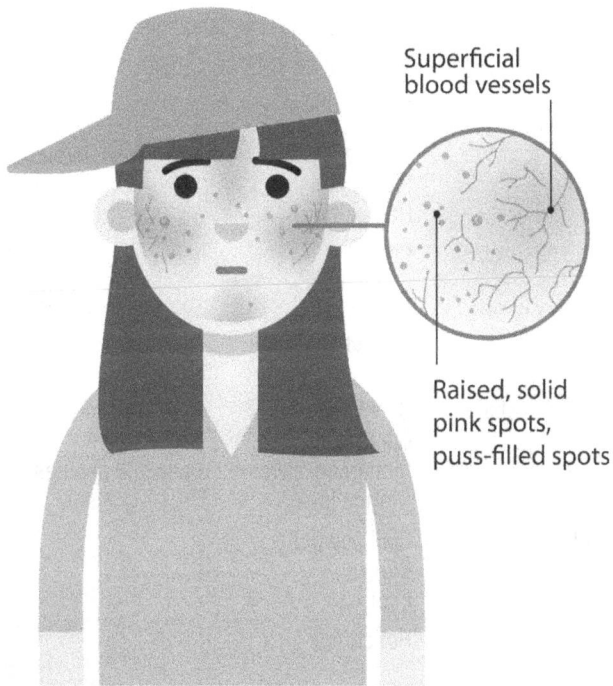

Superficial
blood vessels

Raised, solid
pink spots,
puss-filled spots

Rosacea is a skin disease that can cause flushing, acne, redness—even pain in the face. The nose may become bulbous and even disfigured. The blood vessels in the face and cheeks become enlarged and close to the skin surface. While allergy tends not to play a role in rosacea, food intolerance certainly does. This intolerance tends to be mostly pharmacologic, as many foods that cause dilation of the blood vessels exacerbate the situation. High glycemic foods lead to inflammation and lead to flares of all acne, including rosacea. Below are some examples of irritating foods.

Table 17

Foods That Cause Rosacea Flare-Ups

Foods with capsaicin, which causes dilation of blood vessels	Cayenne peppers Chili peppers Hot peppers Hot sauces Paprika Spicy ketchup
Foods with a high glycemic index	Sugar (all forms - glucose, sucrose, fructose, etc.) High fructose corn syrup Foods sweetened with sugar
Foods that irritate acne	Foods with a high dietary inflammatory index, such as dairy products, milk and cheese (see DII) See foods that worsen acne
Foods with high histamine, which can also dilate blood vessels	Avocado Sauerkraut Chocolate Shellfish Eggplant Strawberries Papaya Tomatoes Pineapple Yogurt Red plums
Foods that are histamine releasers	Citrus Legumes Egg whites Peanuts Eggplant Shellfish Fermented foods Spinach Fish
Foods with cinnamaldehyde, which causes flushing	Chocolate Cinnamon Cinnamon-flavored breads and pastries Orange juice
Foods that are spicy hot	Chili powder Curry Paprika
Foods that are hot in temperature	Hot coffee Hot tea

See Table 20 for resources.

Foods That Can Prevent Rosacea Flares

A healthy diet high in fresh, organic fruits and vegetables, protein, and complex carbohydrates, a small amount of healthy fat, essential fatty acids, and ideally, with minimal refined sugars and processed foods, is a medically sound diet for all patients. This is likewise true for those with rosacea.

Table 18

Foods That Can Prevent Rosacea Flare-Ups	
Foods with diamine oxidase (DAO) blockers (degrades histamine)	Alcohol Black tea Green tea Matcha tea
Supplements known to decrease the inflammation of rosacea	Antioxidants Vitamin A Vitamin E Omega-3 essential fatty acids (we tend to eat more omega-6) Zinc

Adapted from following resources:
Aubdool AA, Brain SD. Neurovascular aspects of skin neurogenic inflammation. *J Investig Dermatol Symp Proc.* 2011 Dec;15(1):33-9. doi: 10.1038/jidsymp.2011.8. PMID: 22076325.
Choi JE, Di Nardo A. Skin neurogenic inflammation. *Semin Immunopathol.* 2018 May;40(3):249-259. doi: 10.1007/s00281-018-0675-z. Epub 2018 Apr 30. PMID: 29713744; PMCID: PMC6047518.
Yuan X, Huang X, Wang B, Huang YX, Zhang YY, Tang Y, Yang JY, Chen Q, Jian D, Xie HF, Shi W, Li J. Relationship between rosacea and dietary factors: A multicenter retrospective case-control survey. *J Dermatol.* 2019 Mar;46(3):219-225. doi: 10.1111/1346-8138.14771. Epub 2019 Jan 18. PMID: 30656725.

Chapter 25

Association of Foods with Obesity and Diabetes: One Person's Meat Is Another Person's Poison

For years now, food allergy consultations have been very common and even in demand in my practice. More and more frequently, some of these patients feel they are gaining weight or having difficulty losing weight due to their food allergy. Having searched the scientific and medical literature thoroughly on behalf of these patients, I can categorically say that food allergy is not directly correlated with diabetes or obesity. However, I have found some associations:

- Allergies, in general, may be associated with diabetes and/or obesity because antihistamines can cause sedation and other side effects that may contribute to obesity for some patients.
- The inflammation of allergy may increase the risk of obesity.
- Many antihistamines have the side effect of increased appetite. For example, cyproheptadine (Periactin) is used to help patients gain weight.
- Excess adipose tissue (meaning excess fat) stimulates release of pro-inflammatory cytokines (hormones of the immune system). The resulting inflammation increases insulin resistance and, therefore, the likelihood of diabetes mellitus, weight gain, and obesity.
- Reduced levels of a hormone known as adiponectin that is increased in chronic inflammation (as well as from excess adipose tissue) is a predictor of cardiovascular mortality and associated with increased fasting glucose, type 2 diabetes, and metabolic abnormalities.

It is my conclusion that it is not so much the foods themselves or even allergy to those foods, but the quality of the diet and effects of excess food consumption, even if the foods are good, clean, and healthy, that puts a patient at risk for diabetes or obesity. The dietary inflammatory index (DII) may also play a role (see Chapter 26).

Glycemic Index

70–100	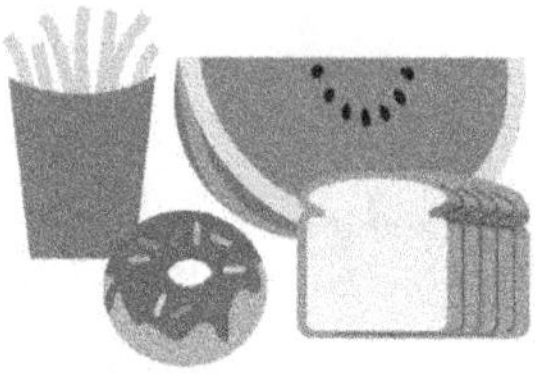 • White wheat bread, donuts, baguette, crackers, waffles • White rice, potatoes, french fries • watermelon • cornflakes
50–70	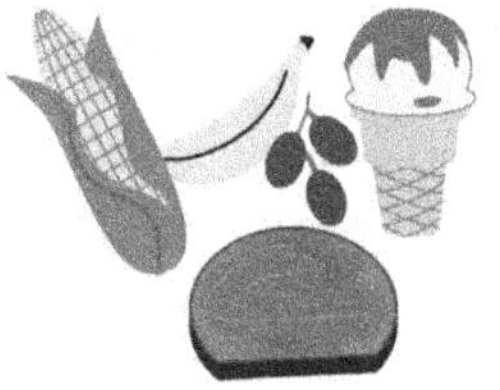 • rye and whole grain bread • corn, couscous, brown rice, spaghetti, popcorn, yams • ice cream, sweet yogurt • banana, grapes
30–50	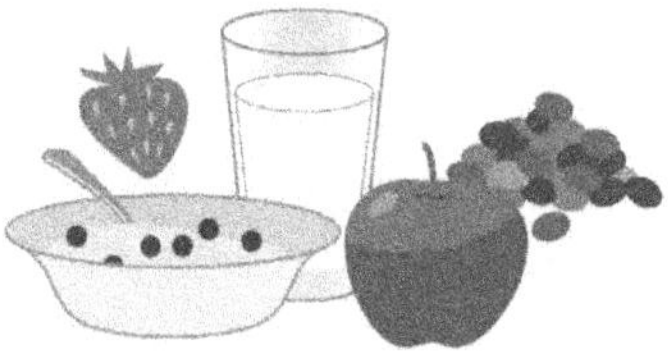 • coarse barley bread • strawberries, apples, oranges • milk and soy milk • natural yogurt • oatmeal, beans
10–30	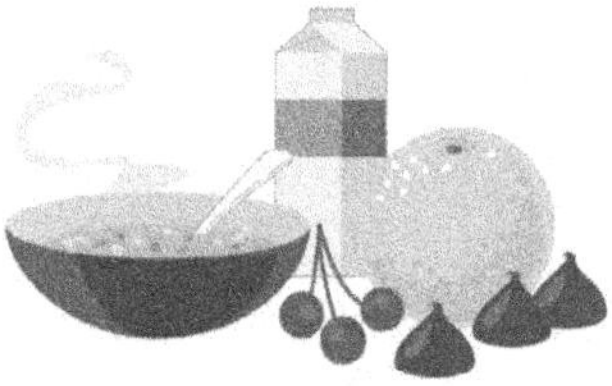 • whole milk • pearled barley, lentils • grapefruit, cherries, apricots • dark 70% chocolate • cashews, walnuts
0–10	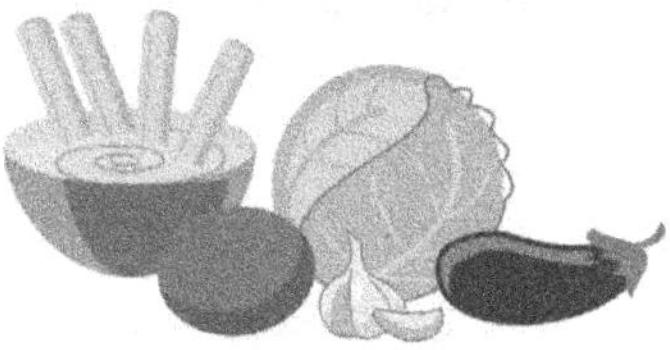 • hummus (chickpeas) • garlic, onion, green pepper • eggplant, broccoli, cabbage, tomatoes, lettuce • mushrooms

Figure 58: The Glycemic Index is an index that rates the degree to which foods affect blood sugar when that food is eaten in isolation. The higher the glycemic index, the greater effect that food has on blood sugar. Conversely, the lower the glycemic index, the less effect that food has on blood sugar.

Recommendations for maintaining a healthy weight

To lose weight and to maintain a healthy weight, the World Health Organization recommends:

1. Decrease sugar, processed food, and carbohydrates in diet.
2. Decrease portions.
3. Participate in 60 minutes of physical activity daily (muscle burns glucose and fat more effectively).
4. Drink more water.
5. Stop smoking, as it increases insulin resistance.
6. Consume fiber to normalize blood sugar and insulin levels.
7. Eat plenty of fresh vegetables.
8. Replace dessert with fresh fruit.
9. Avoid soft drinks and fruit juices.
10. Eat less fast food (concentrated, highly processed, generally low-quality ingredients, high calorie, high glycemic index, and far too easy to grab and eat without thinking about quantities).
11. Eat less in front of the TV or in your car. Intentionally sit and eat.
12. Eat low glycemic index foods (high glycemic index foods increase blood sugar rapidly). (see fig. 58)
13. Get plenty of sleep.

In terms of encouraging an obese child to lose weight, it is far more beneficial for parents to help children overcome obesity if they model healthy behavior, eating habits, and exercise habits as opposed to lecturing, teaching, or punishing. You are your child's best role model. They watch everything you do and model your good behavior (and unfortunately your bad behavior too).

Chapter 26

Taking the "Die" Out of Diet: Obesity and the Dietary Inflammatory Index

The Dietary Inflammatory Index (DII) is an attempt to assign inflammatory points to foods that have a significant impact on health, obesity, and diabetes. The DII was calculated based on inflammatory parameters provoked by the individual foods when consumed in isolation. The health effects of three well-known diets can be seen in detail below.

One study measured inflammation using pro-inflammatory mediators and insulin resistance as markers and correlated them with common dietary patterns and the DII (Hébert 2019). Body mass index and fat mass were correlated with a Western-type diet. On the other hand, inflammatory mediators were inversely related to a healthy dietary pattern.

Overall, using the DII should make it easier and more flexible to have an effective and an anti-inflammatory diet.

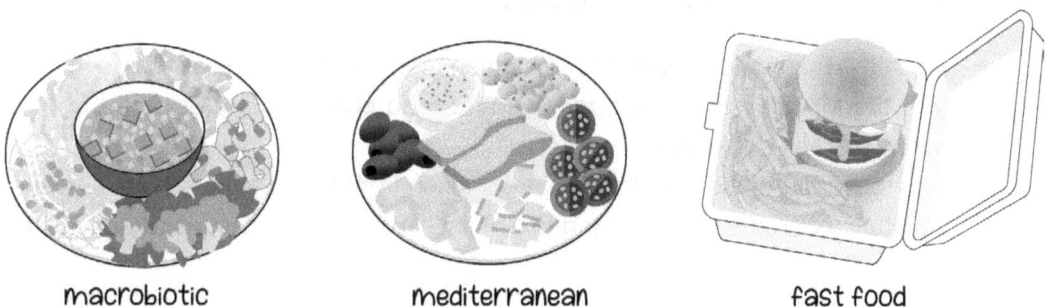

macrobiotic   mediterranean   fast food

Figure 59

Traditional Diet

- Included mainly poultry, fruit, green leafy vegetables, red and organ meat, and hydrogenated fat.
- The positive effect of this diet was thought to be due to higher dietary fiber, vitamin E, folate, and magnesium
- This diet's low glycemic index was related to decreased inflammatory mediators and inversely related to insulin resistance and DII values.

Western Diet

- Higher in saturated fat, high-fat dairy, soft drinks, fruit juices, butter, French fries, pizza, sweets, and processed meat.
- Positively associated with fat mass and BMI.

Fast Food Diet

- Represents typical items on a fast-food menu.
- Clearly an inflammatory diet.

Healthy Diet

- Higher intakes of vegetables and fruit, whole breads and cereals, legumes, eggs, low-fat dairy, and mainly poultry meat.
- Lower consumption of fat and dairy.
- Inversely associated with inflammatory mediators (Hébert 2014).

Mediterranean and Macrobiotic Diets

- Both the macrobiotic and Mediterranean diets are anti-inflammatory.
- For the Mediterranean diet, recipes and food choices were selected from a classic Greek cookbook.
- For the Macrobiotic diet, foods were chosen from the Kushi Institute, a health institute (now closed) dedicated to a holistic macrobiotic lifestyle (Steck 2014).

Anti-Inflammatory Diet

Foods that Fight Inflammation

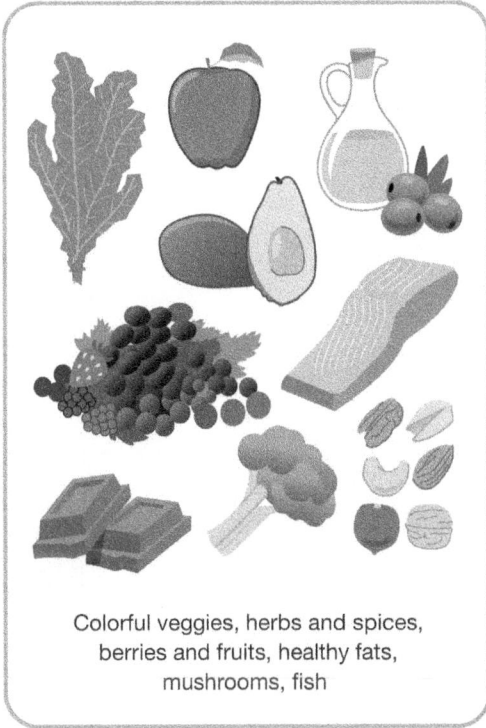

Foods that Cause Inflammation

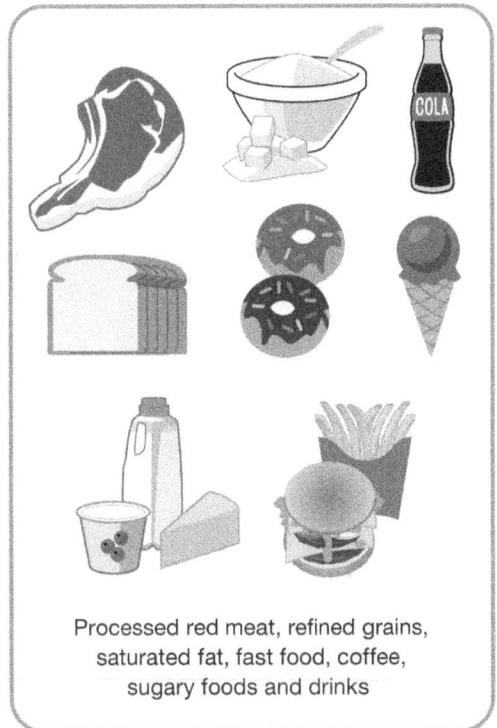

Colorful veggies, herbs and spices,
berries and fruits, healthy fats,
mushrooms, fish

Processed red meat, refined grains,
saturated fat, fast food, coffee,
sugary foods and drinks

Figure 60: Comparison of anti-inflammatory vs. inflammatory foods.

Chapter 27

Just Face It: Facts About Food Allergy and Acne

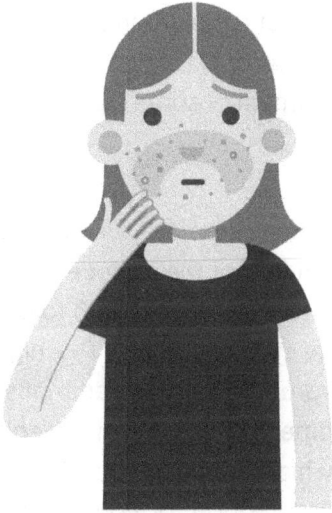

When I was younger and in the middle of yet another acne breakout, my dad would heckle me about eating chocolate. This drove me crazy, as I could not believe chocolate had anything to do with my humiliating situation. As it turns out, he was more correct than either of us could imagine.

The discomfort and embarrassment of acne drives many to consult with an allergist about food allergy. While this is another food association that does not meet the criteria of food allergy, there are definite patterns.

Milk consumption has been implicated in multiple studies and though there seems to be a trend, the studies have failed to prove a dose-response relationship or correlate the response to possible hormones that might be present in the milk of pregnant cows.

The four factors that contribute to acne are: increased sebum production, increased proliferation of follicular skin cells, hormones, and skin bacterial carriage.

Food Nutrients That Can Help Acne

The two most important factors in food validated to affect acne thus far are insulin production and a high glycemic index. A diet high in high glycemic index foods produces spikes in blood glucose and therefore insulin production. As well, insulin increases the body's production of oil, contributing further to acne.

Those who follow a low glycemic diet seem to have fewer acne lesions.

Nutrients That Improve Acne

Low glycemic foods
Vitamin A
Vitamin D
Vitamin E
Antioxidants
Linolenic acid, an essential fatty acid
Linoleic acid, an essential fatty acid
Zinc
Caloric restriction

Vitamins

Derivatives of vitamin A are used to treat acne. Vitamin A in the diet decreases keratinocyte proliferation and has been approved for treatment of acne. Vitamin D and its analogs are used to treat skin cancers, aging, and acne. Vitamin D is known to be anti-proliferative, and analogues of Vitamin D are used in treatment of some skin cancers.

Essential Fatty Acids

The essential (we cannot make them; we need to consume them in our diet) fatty acids of linolenic and linoleic acid are important components of the skin ceramides of the skin barrier. The Western diet consumes a ratio of 10-20:1 of omega-6 to omega-3, whereas a non-Western diet consumption is more typically 2-3:1. The higher ratio is thought to be more pro-inflammatory. In other words, to increase anti-inflammatory benefits of our diet, we need to consume more omega-3 essential fatty acids. It may seem counterintuitive to be consuming fat at all, which seems to be vilified, but think of this as a shift in the types of fat. Some are actually good for you and quite necessary.

In addition, several studies implicate a diet rich in zinc, vitamins A, D, and E, antioxidants, and omega-3 fatty acids may be helpful in reducing acne. These are also thought to be anti-inflammatory in their effect.

If your child really cannot tolerate these supplements in their food form, consider supplementation. However, because some of these nutrients can be toxic and cause problems when over-ingested, it is always important to discuss supplements with your child's doctor in advance.

Chapter 28

Feel No Pain:
Food Allergies are a Trigger for
Migraines and Headaches

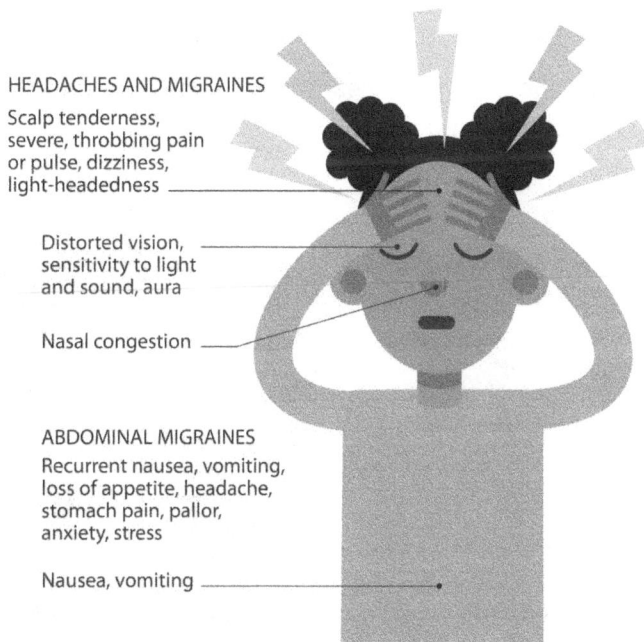

HEADACHES AND MIGRAINES

Scalp tenderness,
severe, throbbing pain
or pulse, dizziness,
light-headedness

Distorted vision,
sensitivity to light
and sound, aura

Nasal congestion

ABDOMINAL MIGRAINES

Recurrent nausea, vomiting,
loss of appetite, headache,
stomach pain, pallor,
anxiety, stress

Nausea, vomiting

As a teenager, I had migraine headaches twice a year, once in the spring and once in the fall. Every season I would forget how severe they had been and when they started again, it would take a lot to convince me I didn't have a brain tumor.

No headache medication would work. I tried nonsteroidal anti-inflammatory medications and acetaminophen. The failure of these traditional pain medications just further validated my assumption that I had a tumor. Finally, on a whim, I tried an antihistamine: it took care of my symptoms in 15 minutes. This was one of my first encounters with allergies.

What Is a Migraine Headache?

I always compare the migraine to an onion; it has multiple layers. Once you get past the first layer, it is a little smaller but it is still there. This is one chronic condition that requires evaluation of all the factors. Moreover, once you eliminate one trigger, it may be easier to determine another pattern, which may reveal another trigger.

Triggering symptoms need to be evaluated. It is certainly much easier to add medication once the inciting causes are removed. In my experience, this can be very frustrating for patients since many have suffered a long time before they find help. Consequently, they want to know right away "the one thing" to avoid or remove from their diet to get rid of the migraine.

My first job when working with migraine patients is to identify and evaluate those substances that trigger their migraines.

What Are the Different Types of Headaches?

My next job is to determine the type of headache. Headaches are broadly divided into migraines, cluster headaches, and tension headaches.

Table 19

Types and Characteristics of Headaches			
Quality of headache	Migraine	Cluster	Tension
Location	Side(s) of head, unilateral or bilateral	Side of head, unilateral, usually centering around one eye	Sides of head, bilateral
Duration	4-72 hours	30-90 minutes, occur in groups over weeks to months	2 hours to days
Severity	Mild to severe	Very severe	Mild to moderate
Aura, or premonitory nausea, sensitivity to light, sound, and odors	Common	No	No
Accompanied by neurologic symptoms such as redness or tearing of the eyes, nasal congestion, or runny nose	Sometimes	Yes	No
Comments	Females>males (2-3:1)	Mostly males	Most common

Adapted from Stanford Medical Health Care. Types of headaches. Stamford Medical website. Updated n.d. Accessed December 12, 2022. https://stanfordhealthcare.org/medical-conditions/brain-and-nerves/headache/types.html.

Children Have Unique Headaches and Migraines

Children can present with interesting forms of headache and migraines. While some children have typical migraine symptoms, others have significant abdominal symptoms with little or no headache whatsoever.

The first time I saw a child with an abdominal migraine, an unusual condition in which a child develops abdominal pain but not head pain, I assessed their environmental and food allergies—but nothing turned up. However, instead of prescribing standard migraine medication, which seems very toxic and is not indicated for children, I searched for an alternative. In the very sparse literature available at that time, I found a relationship between supplementing CoQ10 and carnitine with a decrease in migraine, so that is the direction I headed. While it took a few months, my patient gained control of their headaches and was able to function once again.

Cyclic Vomiting Syndrome is a migraine unique to children that consists of episodes of nausea and vomiting, with no symptoms between episodes. This is a very distressing syndrome and certainly was for one of my young patients until she was on medications.

Causes of Migraine Headaches

Do allergies play a role?

Allergies certainly can be a migraine trigger. For example, when headaches are caused by sinus pain and inflammation, it is very valuable to have a skin test for environmental allergies. Addressing any allergies would also be expected to relieve sinusitis, which can be a comorbid condition that can trigger a migraine or make it more severe.

Food can trigger migraines

Many foods have been implicated in headaches. These foods are thought to be involved in vasodilation or spasm of blood vessels. A four- to eight-week trial of a migraine diet can be helpful in defining food triggers.

Diet and supplementation can help headaches

In terms of diet, supplementation of Coenzyme Q10 (CoQ10), carnitine, magnesium, riboflavin, and cinnamon may be helpful.

- Adherence to the MIND Diet (Mediterranean-DASH Intervention for Neurodegenerative Delay), which features increased vegetables and legumes and decreased refined foods, demonstrated a severe headache decrease of 36%.
- Diets low on the glycemic index have also been shown to reduce migraine headaches.

- Increased intake of omega-3 fatty acids can decrease frequency, duration, and severity of migraine headaches, seemingly related to its anti-inflammatory effect.

IBS may be linked to migraines

Several small studies of only 21 and 30 patients seem to suggest that a food-specific IgG-based elimination diet would be helpful for migraine patients with irritable bowel syndrome. While this is interesting, these studies have yet to be validated in a larger trial.

Testing and Diagnosis

There may be no need to perform any testing. However, if there are neurological symptoms or any warning signs, an MRI of the head or neck or perhaps a full neurologic evaluation may be in order.

Treatment of Migraine Headaches

Are there any conservative treatments for my child?

During an acute attack, nonsteroidal anti-inflammatories and triptans (like sumatriptan) can be used to help stop the headache pain.

While these supplements should only be used under the care of a physician, there is suggestion that Co-enzyme Q10 (ubiquinone) in a dose of 10 mg/kg/day or 200 mg, whichever dose is less, divided twice daily, and carnitine in a dose of 50-100 mg/kg/day, could help with migraines and is reasonably safe for children. This combination has been used for preventing both migraine headaches and a migraine unique to children known as Abdominal Migraine or Cyclic Vomiting Syndrome.

Other preventative treatments include the supraorbital nerve stimulator, vagus nerve stimulator, and the transcranial magnetic stimulator. Cognitive behavioral therapy has also proven useful in preventing and stopping migraines.

Prevention should also include proper hydration, stress reduction, diet, and exercise.

My approach to helping a neurologist treat migraines is to help identify as many triggers as possible. Migraine triggers tend to be multi-layered and the discovery process is like peeling an onion. The more triggers you resolve, the easier it is to identify the pattern and complete the elimination process. Therefore, careful identification of the circumstances surrounding migraines, keeping a journal, and elimination of allergies and other triggers is critical.

When is a headache not just a headache?

In rare cases, a migraine may signal a severe medical condition such as a brain tumor, aneurysm, or stroke. The following warning signs signal that the headache is not just a headache but could be a sign of something serious. When your child feels a migraine coming on, the first question you should ask yourself is, *Are any warning signs present?*

Migraine headache warning signs

- It appears suddenly, is more severe and different from past headaches, or worsens over time.
- It is triggered by exertion, coughing, or bending.
- It is linked with a stiff neck and fever.
- It is accompanied by disturbed vision or speech or numbness, tingling, or weakness in a part of the body.
- It makes it difficult for you to think and remember.
- It causes severe vomiting.
- It follows a head injury.
- It starts after age 50.

Tracking triggers: Check each item on the list in Table 20 on the next page that seems to bring on your child's migraines.

Table 20

Tracking Migraine Triggers		
Categories of Triggers	**Examples**	

Dietary Factors	Alcoholic beverages
	Artificial sweeteners
	Beans
	Caffeine (excess, withdrawal)
	Chocolate
	Citrus fruits
	Dairy products
	Fatty foods
	Nuts
	Onions
	Sour cream
		Yeast extracts
		Yogurt
		Food additives:
		    Monosodium glutamate (MSG)
		    Nitrites (e.g., in hot dogs,
		    deli meats)
		Foods containing tyramine:
		    Aged cheeses
		    Chianti wine
		    Dried and smoked meat
		    Pickled herring

Environmental Factors	Air pollution Bright light Complex visual patterns (lined shirts) Environmental allergies Flickering light sources Fluorescent lighting Fumes from industrial complexes	Motion Perfumes Secondhand cigarette smoke Strong odors Travel Weather changes
Hormonal Factors	Birth-control pills Estrogen blockers Estrogen replacement Giving birth Menopause	Menses Pregnancy Puberty Testosterone Testosterone blockers
Lifestyle Factors	Cigarette smoking Dehydration Disrupted sleep patterns Fatigue Irregular eating habits Stress	
Medications	Blood pressure medications Diuretics Drugs that dilate blood vessels (sildenafil, nitroglycerine) Medications with hormones Pain medications that are used too frequently Vitamins	
Physical Factors	Arthritis of neck Exertion	Head trauma Invasive medical tests

Adapted from the following resources:
Stanford Medical Health Care. Types of headaches. Stamford Medical website. Updated n.d. Accessed December 12, 2022. https://stanfordhealthcare.org/medical-conditions/brain-and-nerves/headache/types.html
American Migraine Foundation. Top ten migraine triggers and how to deal with them. American Migraine Foundation website. Updated n.d. Accessed December 12, 2022. https://americanmigrainefoundation.org/resource-library/top-10-migraine-triggers/.

Chapter 29

Feeding the Protector: Food Allergy and Immunodeficiencies

Food allergy, for unknown reasons, is also associated with several immunodeficiency syndromes. Primary immunodeficiency diseases are genetic diseases that impair normal functioning of the immune system, causing a pattern of increased and recurrent infections, typically with unusual microorganisms that are trivial for an intact immune system to defend against.

IPEX Syndrome (immunodysregulation, polyendocrinopathy, enteropathy, X-linked) typically presents at three to four months old. The incidence is one in 1.6 million children (Bonilla 2015). IPEX is associated with severe enteropathy with small bowel atrophy (like celiac disease), diabetes, thyroid disease, and decreases in red blood cells, platelets, and cells of the immune system known as neutrophils. It is associated with increased rates of eczema and IgE-mediated food allergies, as well as non-IgE-mediated food allergies such as FPIES (see Chapter 18).

Dock 8 deficiency is associated with recurrent pulmonary and viral skin infections, high IgE levels, and increased risk of many infections due to immunodeficiency as well as increased risk of malignancies. There is a high rate of asthma, eczema, and IgE-mediated food allergies. Dock 8 deficiency presents around age 12 and is exceedingly rare, estimated to affect 1 in one million patients (Bonilla 2015).

Netherton Syndrome causes immunodeficiency and increased infections, especially skin infections and upper respiratory tract infections, severe dermatitis, bamboo hair, and red, scaly skin known as erythroderma, as well as high frequency of allergic rhinitis, food allergy, and asthma. Netherton syndrome presents at birth and is thought to affect 1 in 200,000 newborns.

Wiskott-Aldrich Syndrome is characterized by low platelets, immunodeficiency and frequent infections, increased risk of autoimmune disease, increased risk of malignancy, and increased eczema in patients with more severe forms of the disease. The prevalence is 1-10 cases per one million males (females are carriers and therefore do not get the disease but can pass the disease on to their offspring) (Bonilla 2015). On average, it presents from birth to 25 years old (Bonilla 2015).

IgA deficiency is the most common of the primary immunodeficiency syndromes and usually one of the least severe. Patients have an increased risk of sinopulmonary infections and autoimmunity as well as allergic conditions, including allergic rhinitis, allergic conjunctivitis, allergic urticaria, eczema, asthma, and food allergies. The prevalence of IgA deficiency is 1 in 223 to 1 in 1000 people and it typically presents after about four years old (Bonilla 2015).

Most of these syndromes involve very serious immunodeficiencies that should be managed by a board-certified allergist-immunologist.

Chapter 30

Don't Bring Me Down: Food and Depression

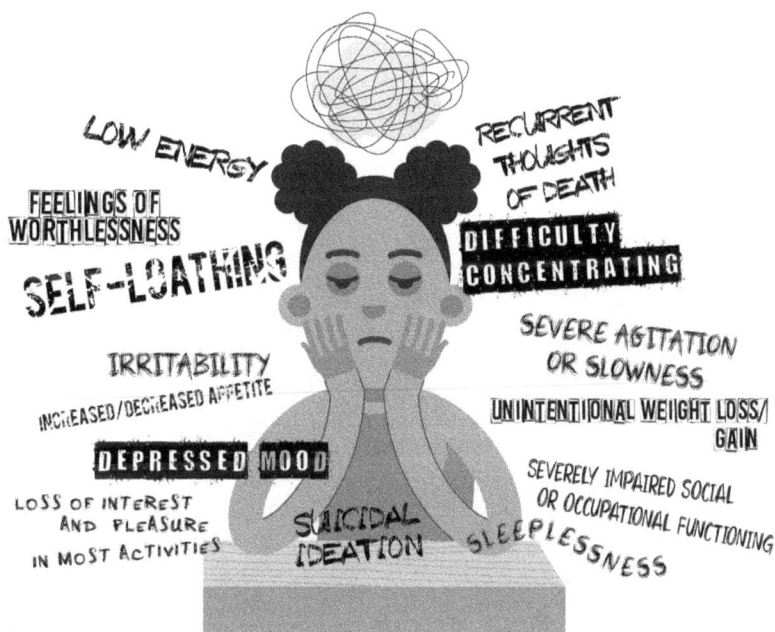

Whereas a diet with a relatively low dietary inflammatory index was associated with a lower incidence of depression symptoms (odds ratio=0.81) in a non-dose dependent way, a high-quality diet, regardless of the specific one, was associated with lower risk of depressive symptoms over time in a dose-responsive fashion (odds ratio 0.64-0.78 responding in a dose-dependent way). Fish and vegetables alone were also associated with a lower risk of depression (odds ratio 0.86 and 0.82, respectively).

A diet that reduced the risk of depression was characterized as one with a high intake of fruit, vegetables, whole grains, fish, olive oil, low-fat dairy, and antioxidants and low in animal foods—also called a low dietary inflammatory index (Hébert 2019). On the other hand, a diet in which red or processed meat, refined grains, sweets, butter, high-fat gravies, dairy products, potatoes, and low intake of foods such as fruits and vegetables—the typical Western diet (see fig. 58)—was associated with an increased risk of depression (Hébert 2019, Molendijk 2017).

Conclusion

Thank you for taking this journey with me through food allergy, intolerance, and toxicity. My hope is that I have made these complicated medical concepts understandable and helpful for you and your family and that you are now better informed if any of these issues apply to you or your children.

While allergy is a much bigger and more complicated field than most people understand, there is an entire medical specialty dedicated to helping you and your children—the allergist-immunologist. Because of the extensive training we receive, allergist-immunologists are also able to differentiate between allergy and intolerance in most cases and are well-versed in the latest solutions and state-of-the-art treatments.

Then there is toxicity… If we as humans living on our beautiful planet Earth do not act, we will all be affected by toxicity in one form or another in the future. This is an unfortunate side effect of the way our food is farmed, processed, prepared, stored, and packaged. By producing a large amount of food for our Earth's growing population, we have selected efficiencies that are not entirely benign.

It is time to pause and consider how those choices may affect us now and in the future.

I wish you and your family good health.

Kindest regards,
Julie Wendt, MD

Appendix

Finding a Board-Certified Allergist-Immunologist

Only the Best for Your Child

Your child deserves to have a physician who is board-certified in Allergy and Immunology when you are looking for testing and treatment of these diseases. A board-certified allergist-immunologist has undergone rigorous training in Internal Medicine and/or Pediatrics, a fellowship in Allergy and Immunology, and must pass licensure boards in Internal Medicine and/or Pediatrics and Allergy and Immunology. Continuous medical education and testing ensure your child's allergist-immunologist stays current in this constantly changing field.

You can find a local board-certified allergist-immunologist at The American Board of Allergy and Immunology website at abai.org.

Anaphylaxis Action Plan

ANAPHYLAXIS ACTION PLAN

Name _____ Date _____ Triggers to Avoid_____

Become familiar with your Anaphylaxis Action Plan before a crisis arises. Ask questions of your Allergist now. I highly recommended that you have—at minimum—an annual in-office review with your Allergist to review your Anaphylaxis Action Plan and practice using your epinephrine auto-injector. Your Allergist will adjust your Anaphylaxis Action Plan periodically based on your symptoms.

Green Zone - GO

Green Zone Symptoms

You are completely well and not experiencing any symptoms.

Taking Green Zone medications on a regular basis is only necessary when the causes and triggers of anaphylaxis are unknown or your symptoms are unpredictable.

Green Zone medications and instructions

1. Take your non-sedating anti-H1 histamine daily.
2. Take your anti-H2 histamine daily.
3. Take your sedating antihistamine as needed at night.
4. Take your anti-leukotriene by mouth at bedtime.
5. Carry your epinephrine pen with you everywhere. Always keep it with you, know how to use it, and know when it expires.

Yellow Zone - CAUTION

Yellow Zone Symptoms

You are starting to experience symptoms: minor hives, lip swelling, flushing without dizziness, itching but NO chest pain, shortness of breath, swelling of the throat, or tongue or airway compromise.

Yellow Zone medications and instructions

1. Take all of your regular medication as usual.
2. Take an extra dose of your non-sedating anti-H1 histamine and anti-H2 histamine daily.
3. Take a steroid as directed by your Allergist-Immunologist.
4. If you are asthmatic and/or wheeze, use rescue inhaler.
5. Carry your epinephrine pen with you everywhere. Always keep it with you, know how to use it, and know when it expires.

Get ready for a possible increase in anaphylactic symptoms

1. Find your epinephrine auto-injector and have it ready in case you need it.
2. If you are away from help (hiking, on a mountain, in a remote area), stay calm but call for help immediately.
3. If you are in a remote location and any symptoms begin to escalate, consider using your epinephrine pen immediately and move towards help.

Red Zone - STOP

Red Zone Symptoms

You are now experiencing airway compromise (swelling of the throat or tongue), dizziness (which can be a sign of low blood pressure), hives all over your body, chest pain, shortness of breath, wheezing, and/or a feeling of impending doom.

Red Zone medications and instructions

1. Find your epinephrine pen if you don't already have it.
2. Use your epinephrine pen immediately. It should have an effect within 15 seconds to 2 minutes. If it does not take effect, your symptoms worsen, or you begin to lose consciousness, use your second epinephrine pen. If you are asthmatic, use your rescue inhaler.
3. While you are treating yourself, CALL 9-1-1.
4. If you can swallow without choking, take an extra dose of your non-sedating anti-H1 histamine and anti-H2 histamine and a steroid, if you have one. If you cannot swallow, do not try to take your medication until your throat symptoms relieve with epinephrine.

©2022 Julie A. Wendt

Download this form by clicking the QR Code or visiting
https://relieveallergyaz.com/anaphylaxis

Asthma Action Plan

ASTHMA ACTION PLAN

Name _____ Date _____ Best Peak Flow_____

Green Zone - GO

Green Zone Symptoms

- Peak Flow is ≥80% of personal best peak flow.
- You are completely well and not experiencing any asthma symptoms.

When no Peak Flow test is available, you should meet the following standards:

- You show no symptoms of asthma, you're able to perform your usual activities of daily living, exercise without compromise, sleep without difficulty.
- You have used a rescue inhaler less than once per week during the day, and less than twice per month during the night (being awakened from your sleep) or first thing in the morning upon awakening. Alternately, no unexpected increase in rescue inhaler use.

Green Zone medications and instructions

1. Continue regular use of maintenance medication as prescribed.
2. Use your rescue inhaler as needed to relieve shortness of breath, wheezing, chest tightness, or cough related to asthma. (If use increases to twice a day or more unscheduled or twice per month use on awakening, upgrade to the Yellow Zone.)
3. If you have a component of exertional asthma, you may premedicate with 1-2 puffs of your rescue medication 20 minutes prior to exercise. This use doesn't necessarily reflect a worsening of asthma.

Yellow Zone - CAUTION

Yellow Zone Symptoms

- Peak Flow is between 60-80% of personal best peak flow.
- Asthma symptoms are beginning or you are being exposed to your typical triggers.

When no Peak Flow test is available, you may have these symptoms:

- You may be short of breath, wheezing, coughing, or have chest tightness.
- Your use of rescue medication exceeds your normal usage; two or more unscheduled daytime uses during a typical week or two or more unscheduled uses per month upon awakening during the nighttime or early morning.

Yellow Zone medications and instructions

1. Continue preventive medication as prescribed.
2. When needed to control shortness of breath, wheezing, or coughing due to asthma, take your rescue inhaler as directed or take your rescue medication through your nebulizer. If use is required more frequently than instructed (usually 4 hours), upgrade status to Red Zone and follow those instructions.
3. Schedule a follow up appointment with me or your Allergist-Immunologist as soon as possible.
4. Now is the time to add steroids or added rescue medication as instructed by your allergist.
5. Repeat Peak Flow test and/or reassess symptoms every few hours. If necessary, step up or down to the appropriate zone and follow those instructions.

Red Zone - STOP

Red Zone Symptoms

Peak Flow is ≤60%.

- Symptoms are shortness of breath, wheezing, coughing, chest tightness.
- Your rescue medication does not work effectively for 4 hours and the length of time it is effective is steadily decreasing.
- You are having thoughts such as, "I need to be in the emergency room" or a feeling of doom.

Red Zone medications and instructions

1. Go to the emergency room.
2. On the way to the ER:
   a. Take your rescue medication.
   b. If you have airway impairment and you have been given an epinephrine auto-injector, use it.
   c. Take a steroid in the recommended dose if you have it and you can swallow properly.
3. Make an appointment with your Allergist-Immunologist as soon as you are released from the emergency room.

©2022 Julie A. Wendt

Download this form by clicking the QR Code or visiting
https://relieveallergyaz.com/asthma

RECIPES FOR INCREASING FOOD TOLERANCE
for children allergic to raw milk and egg

The intent of these recipes is to aid the child to increase their tolerance of and, ideally, outgrow their milk and egg allergies by consuming baked milk and baked egg products regularly, but only if the child tolerates them *with no symptoms whatsoever*. Following are recipes that parents and caregivers can make and feed the allergic child if the Allergist-Immunologist believes they may be allergic and this technique would help.

Jam-Topped Muffins
for increasing tolerance of raw milk

Yield
Makes twelve 3-inch muffins
1 muffin = 1/12 cup milk = about 0.66-0.73 g milk per muffin

Ingredients
1 cup 2% milk (8 fluid ounces/8.8 grams of milk)
2 tablespoons canola or other vegetable oil
1 large egg* (if allergic to egg, use egg replacement equivalent)
1 teaspoon vanilla extract
1¼ cups all-purpose flour (may substitute almond or rice flour, depending on child's allergies)
½ cup sugar
2 teaspoons baking powder
¼ teaspoon salt

Directions
1. Preheat oven to 350 degrees F. Line standard-size muffin pans with muffin/cupcake liners.
2. Whisk together the liquid ingredients: milk, canola oil, egg or egg replacement, and vanilla extract. Set aside.
3. In a separate bowl, mix the flour, sugar, baking powder, and salt.
4. Add the liquid ingredients to the dry ingredients and stir until combined.
5. Pour the mixture into the muffin liners, dividing equally and using ALL the batter.
6. Bake for 30-35 minutes (NOT LESS).
7. Top with small amount of jam or jelly, to taste.

Recipe Notes
Follow this recipe exactly and use all the batter.
Bake at the temperature and time recommended to be sure milk is fully baked.
Follow instructions for egg allergy (*) if needed.
Make standard-sized muffins (3-inch diameter) using either one 12-muffin pan or two 6-muffin pans. DO NOT use jumbo or mini muffin pans.

Banana or Applesauce Muffins
for increasing tolerance of raw egg

Yield

Makes six 3-inch muffins
One 3-inch muffin = 1/3 egg = about 2.2 grams baked egg

Ingredients

2 tablespoons cow's milk*
  (if allergic to milk, use soy, rice, or almond milk)
¼ cup canola or other vegetable oil
1 cup mashed ripe banana or applesauce
2 eggs
½ teaspoon vanilla extract
1 cup all-purpose flour (may substitute almond or rice flour, depending on child's allergies)
1/3 cup sugar
1 teaspoon baking powder
¼ teaspoon salt
¼ teaspoon cinnamon

Directions

1. Preheat oven to 350 degrees F. Line a standard-size muffin pan with
   six muffin/cupcake liners.
2. Whisk together the liquid ingredients: milk or milk substitute, canola oil,
   mashed banana or applesauce, eggs, and vanilla extract. Set aside.
3. In a separate bowl, mix the flour or flour substitute, sugar, baking powder, salt,
   and cinnamon.
4. Add the liquid ingredients to the dry ingredients and stir until combined.
   Some small lumps may remain.
5. Pour the mixture into the muffin liners, dividing equally and using ALL the batter.
6. Bake 30 to 35 minutes or until golden brown and firm to touch.

Recipe Notes

Follow this recipe exactly and use all the batter.
Bake at the temperature and time recommended to be sure egg is fully baked.
Follow instructions for milk allergy (*) if needed.
Make standard-sized muffins (3-inch diameter) using one 6-muffin pan.
DO NOT use jumbo or mini muffin pans.

Can Food Cause Cancer?

One in every two men and one in every three women in the United States will develop cancer at some point in their lifetime (ACS 2010).

Two intergovernmental agencies, the National Toxicology Program (NTP) (Department of Health and Human Services) and the International Agency for Research on Cancer (IARC) (World Health Organization), conduct and coordinate research into the causes of cancer. They also collect and publish surveillance data regarding the occurrence of cancer worldwide.

Annually, the HHS publishes the NTP's Report on Carcinogens, the result of their ongoing research of chemical, physical, and biological agents, mixtures, and exposure circumstances that are known or reasonably anticipated to cause cancer in humans. It then labels them as either known human carcinogen or reasonably anticipated to be a human carcinogen, as follows:

On the next 12 pages is a summary of agents that are "known human carcinogens" or "reasonably anticipated to be a human carcinogen" and that can currently be found in foods, the foods with the highest concentration, and potential side effects. Many agents have been found, such as benzidine in food dyes, and banned because of being listed by the NTP or IARC. As they are no longer permitted in foods, they do not make the list.

Group 1 chemicals are "known human carcinogens" for IARC whereas NTP uses terminology "known to be human carcinogens" in its report; Group 2a chemicals are classified as "reasonably anticipated to be a human carcinogen" by IARC and NTP prefers "reasonably anticipated to be human carcinogens." As these are two independent agencies, they do not necessarily conduct studies on the same chemicals. Therefore, if a chemical is not listed under both agencies, it is not necessarily a failure to acknowledge the danger of the substance.

Table 21

Substances in our Food Supply that are Known Carcinogens or Reasonably	
Carcinogen	**Found in these foods**
Acetaldehyde	Wine, yogurt, fruit juice, pureed fruit, baby food, preserved vegetables, soy sauce, vinegar, fermented foods
Acrylamide	French fries, potato chips; crackers, bread, cookies, breakfast cereals, canned black olives, prune juice, coffee; fried and roasted foods
Aflatoxins	Corn, nuts, cottonseed, peanuts
Alcoholic beverages	Alcoholic beverages
2-amino-3,4-dimethylimidazo [4,5-f] quinoline (MelQ)	Temperature-cooked meats, sardines, beef, and hamburger
2-amino-3,8 dimethylimidazo [4,5-f] quinoxaline (MelQx)	Temperature-cooked meats, sardines, beef, and hamburger
2-amino-3-methylimidazo [4,5-f] quinoline (IQ)	Temperature-cooked meats, sardines, beef, and hamburger
2-amino-1-methyl-6-phenylimidazo [4,5-b] pyridine (PhiP)	Temperature-cooked meats, sardines, beef, and hamburger
Androgenic steroids	Meat, poultry, pork and fish
Areca nut	Chewed as a stimulant, with or without tobacco
Aristolochic acid	Wild ginger, "traditional medicines", ingredient in dietary supplements
Arsenic	Drinking water, seafood, rice, rice cereals, mushroom, poultry, some fruit juices
Benzene	Soft drinks, meat, butter, eggs, fruits, butter
Benz[a]anthracene	Charcoal-broiled, barbecued, and smoked meats, roasted coffee, vegetable oils, baker's yeast and creosote
Benz[b]fluoroanthene	Charcoal-grilled and smoked meats, especially pork, beef, and sausage, trace levels in grain food, Charcoal-grilled vegetables
Benz[j]fluoroanthene, Benz[k]fluoroanthene	Grilled and charred meats
Benzo(a)pyrene	Smoked and charcoal-grilled meats, especially pork, beef, sausage, trace amounts in grain foods
Beryllium	Raw carrots, corn, water, food grown in soil
Betel, with or without tobacco	Chewed as a stimulant, with or without tobacco

Table 21 continued

Anticipated to be Human Carcinogens		
Effects on humans	IARC	NTP
"Hangover"; rapid heart rate, headache, upset stomach, memory impairment, irreversible DNA damage, breast, liver, and oral cancer	1	2a
DNA mutations, ovarian and endometrial cancer	2a	2a
Hepatotoxicity, cancer, immunosuppression, liver cancer	1	1
Liver cancer (see also acetaldehyde, a byproduct of alcohol), alcohol increases solubility and aids absorption of other toxins	1	1
Reasonably anticipated to be a human carcinogen		2a
Reasonably anticipated to be a human carcinogen		2a
Reasonably anticipated to be a human carcinogen		2a
Reasonably anticipated to be a human carcinogen		2a
Liver damage, liver cancer, hepatitis		
Mouth and oral cancer; stimulant, euphoria, flushing, high blood pressure, heart rate, and palpitations; sweating, nausea, vomiting, diarrhea, dizziness, heart disease, dependence; use with tobacco greatly increases risk of oral cancers	1	
Nephrotoxic, kidney, bladder, and urinary tract cancers	1	1
Congenital defects, cognitive development abnormality, cardiovascular disease, diabetes, poisoning, and death; bladder and skin cancer		1
Drowsiness, dizziness, rapid or irregular heartbeat, headaches, tremors, confusion, unconsciousness, death (at high levels), leukemia and lymphoma, multiple myeloma		1
Reasonably anticipated to be a human carcinogen		2a
Reasonably anticipated to be a human carcinogen		2a
Reasonably anticipated to be a human carcinogen		2a
Irritation, rash, burning, skin, and lung cancer, pancreatic, prostate, stomach and colorectal cancer, type 2 diabetes	1	2a
Beryllium sensitization, chronic beryllium disease; may affect lung, liver, kidneys, heart, nervous and lymphatic system; dyspnea, weakness, fatigue, loss of appetite, weight loss, joint pain, cough, fever		1
Mouth and oral cancer, stimulant, euphoria, flushing, high blood pressure, heart rate, and palpitations, sweating, nausea, vomiting, diarrhea, dizziness, heart disease, dependence; use with tobacco greatly increases risk of oral cancers	1	

Table 21 continued

Substances in our Food Supply that are Known Carcinogens or Reasonably	
Carcinogen	**Found in these foods**
Bromodichloremethane	Drinking water
1,3-Butadiene	Drinking water, food
Butylated hydroxyanisole (BHA)	Butter, lard, meats, cereals, baked goods, sweets, beer, vegetable oils, potato chips, snack foods, nuts and nut products, dehydrated potatoes, and flavoring agents
Cadmium	Cereals, vegetables, nuts, starchy roots and potatoes, meat and meat products, vegetable oils, seeds
Chlorinated paraffins	Contaminated food
Chloroform	Contaminated food and drinking water
Chromium	Meats, grains, nuts, spices, fruits, vegetables, beer, wine, and brewer's yeast
Clonorchis sinensis, Chinese liver fluke	Raw and undercooked fish
Creosote, coal tar	Smoked meats
p-Cresidine	Contaminant in Red #40
Danthron (1,8-dihydroxyanthraquinone)	Rhubarb root, senna leaf and pod, cascara
DDT (4,4'-Dichlorodiphenyl-trichloroethane)	Meat, fish, dairy, vegetables
Diazinon	Drinking water, contaminated food
Diazoaminobenzene	Additive contaminant in foods
Dibenz[a,h]anthracene	Smoked and barbecued foods
Dibenzo[a,e]pyrene and Dibenzo[a,h]pyrene	Charcoal grilled, barbecued, broiled, smoked and fried meats and foods
Dibenzo[a,l]pyrene	Charcoal-grilled and smoked meats, especially pork, beef and sausage, trace amount in grains
1,2-Dibromo-3-chloropropane (DBCP)	Nematicide and soil contaminant in food and water
1,2-Dibromoethane (ethylene dibromide)	Pesticide contaminant of food and drinking water
1,4-Dichlorobenzene	Pesticide contaminant of food and drinking water
3,3'-Dichlorobenzidine and its dihydrochloride	Fish
Dichloromethane (Methylene chloride)	Food additive used to process spices and beer hops, remove caffeine from coffee and tea; de-greener for citrus, dilutes color additives for fruits and vegetables

Table 21 continued

Anticipated to be Human Carcinogens

Effects on humans	IARC	NTP
Reasonably anticipated to be a human carcinogen		2a
Damage to the central nervous system, blurred vision, decreased blood pressure, headache, nausea, fainting, fatigue; leukemia, carcinogenic		1
Reasonably anticipated to be a human carcinogen		2a
Nausea, vomiting, stomach cramps, diarrhea, kidney damage, fragile bones, death, lung, prostate, kidney, pancreatic, breast and urinary cancer	1	1
Reasonably anticipated to be a human carcinogen		2a
Hepatotoxicity, nephrotoxicity; reasonably anticipated to be a human carcinogen		2a
Skin irritation, headaches, dizziness, nausea, impaired judgement and coordination, mood change, nephrotoxic, hepatotoxic; lung, sinus and nasopharyngeal cancer	1	1
Biliary infections, stones, and cancer, hepatotoxic, eosinophilia, fever, chills, itch, abdominal pain, malaise, liver cancer (cholangiocarcinoma)	1	
Skin and scrotal cancer	2a	
Immune system tumors		2a
Reasonably anticipated to be a human carcinogen		2a
Vomiting, tremors, shakiness, seizures; hepatotoxic, can affect reproduction; reasonably anticipated to be a human carcinogen	2a	2a
Central nervous system toxicity, stomach pain, vomiting, diarrhea, runny nose, watery eyes, drooling, loss of appetite, associated with lung cancer in some studies	2a	
Reasonably anticipated to be a human carcinogen		2a
Irritation of skin and eyes; probable human carcinogen	2a	2a
Reasonably anticipated to be a human carcinogen		2a
Probable human carcinogen	2a	2a
Reasonably anticipated to be a human carcinogen		2a
Reasonably anticipated to be a human carcinogen		2a
Weight loss, immunosuppression, hepatitis, diarrhea, tremors, and seizures; reasonably anticipated to be a human carcinogen		2a
Reasonably anticipated to be a human carcinogen		2a
Slight vision and hearing impairment, burns of throat, stomach, may be neurotoxic, may be cardiotoxic; probable human carcinogen	2a	2a

Table 21 continued

Substances in our Food Supply that are Known Carcinogens or Reasonably

Carcinogen	Found in these foods
Dieldrin	Contaminated root crops, fish & seafood
Di(2-ethylyhexyl) phthalate	Contaminated meat, fat, cereals, fruit, vegetables, milk and dairy products
Dimethylcarbamoyl chloride	Contaminated foods
Dimethyl sulfate	Additive to impart savory flavor; beetroot, asparagus, cabbage, corn, and seafoods when cooked
Dimethylvinyl chloride	Vinyl chloride can leach from plastic PVC bottles or containers used to contain foods or beverages; amount limited in packaging
Epstein-Barr Virus (EBV) infection	Contaminated foods or drinks (body fluids)
Estrogen	Red and processed meats, refined grains, processed foods
Ethanol in alcoholic beverages	Alcoholic beverages
Ethyl carbamate (urethane)	Soy sauce, kimchi, breads, wine and saki, alcoholic beverages
Ethylene thiourea	Found in fresh, frozen and baked food products (fruit, vegetables, canned goods and soups), beverages (milk, juice and beer) and water where it is believed to be a metabolite of ethylene bisdithiocarbamate (EBDC) fungicides
N-Ethyl-N-nitrosourea	Food treated with nitrates for coloring, flavoring or preservation; processed fish and meat
Formaldehyde	Fruits and vegetables, meats, fish, shellfish, dried mushrooms
Furan	Thermally processed canned or jarred foods as soups, sauces, beans, pasta meals, and baby foods, coffee that is roasted
Glycidol	Infant formula and margarine
Glyphosate	Bagels, honey, eggs, flour, and infant formula
Helicobacter pylori (infection)	Contaminated foods or drinks (saliva)
Hexachlorobenzene	Fish, fish and vegetable oils, pumpkin seeds
Hexachloroethane	Contaminated food and drinking water
Indeno[1,2,3-cd] pyrene	Shellfish, especially mussels and oysters, cooked meat
Isoprene	Carrots, sweet oranges, and wild carrots
Isopropyl alcohol	Food flavorings, fragrances, preservatives, colorants, and sweeteners, soft drinks

Table 21 continued

Anticipated to be Human Carcinogens		
Effects on humans	**IARC**	**NTP**
Malaise, incoordination, headache, dizziness, gastrointestinal disturbances, seizures, probable human carcinogen	2a	
Reasonably anticipated to be a human carcinogen		2a
Damage to mucous membranes of nose, throat, lungs, can cause shortness of breath, probable human carcinogen	2a	2a
Damages liver, kidneys, heart and central nervous system, blisters skin; probable human carcinogen	2a	2a
Reasonably anticipated to be a human carcinogen		2a
Mononucleosis, fever, chills, lymphadenopathy, fatigue, hepatomegaly, splenomegaly, sore throat; nasopharyngeal and stomach cancer and lymphomas (Burkitt's lymphoma and Hodgkin's lymphoma)	1	1
Breast cancer, colorectal cancer	1	1
Liver cancer (see also acetaldehyde, byproduct), assists solubility and other toxins	1	
Headache, nausea, vomiting, dizziness, syncope, toxic to brain and bone marrow; probable human carcinogen	2a	
Reasonably anticipated to be a human carcinogen		2a
Increased rate of brain tumors (gliomas), colorectal, bladder, and breast cancers; neurodevelopmental disorders such as autism, dyslexia, and ADHD	2a	
Nausea, vomiting, diarrhea, abdominal pain, pain and burning of the esophagus, shortness of breath, fatigue, myeloid cancer, cancer of sinuses and nasopharynx	1	1
Reasonably anticipated to be a human carcinogen		2a
Skin and mucous membrane and respiratory tract irritant; CNS depression and stimulant; probable human carcinogen	2a	2a
Possible effect on microbiome, skin and eye irritation; probable human carcinogen	2a	
Ulcers, abdominal pain, gastric cancer	1	
High levels may cause adverse effects on the nervous system such as weakness, tremors, and convulsions; skin sores; and liver and thyroid effects; cause damage to the liver and reproductive system and can cause developmental effects		2a
Reasonably anticipated to be a human carcinogen		2a
Reasonably anticipated to be a human carcinogen		2a
Reasonably anticipated to be a human carcinogen		2a
Dizziness, low blood pressure, nausea, stomach pain, increased heart rate, slurred speech, respiratory depression; laryngeal and sinus cancer	1	

Table 21 continued

Substances in our Food Supply that are Known Carcinogens or Reasonably

Carcinogen	Found in these foods
IQ (2-amino-3-methylimidazo[4,5-f] quinolonine)	Smoked and cooked meats
Kepone (chlordecone)	Fish, shellfish, banana peels
Lead	Candy, baby foods, cookies and teething biscuits, chocolate, peas, sweet potatoes, mustard greens, other vegetables
Lindane (hexachlorocyclohexane and isomers)	Pretreated seeds, including sunflowers, peas, wheat, barley and oats
Magenta	Colorings
5-Methoxypsoralen	Parsnips and celery, in bergamot and lime oils, and in derivative products
Methyleugenol	Anise, nutmeg, mace, pixuri seeds, basil, blackberry essence, bananas, walnuts, citrus, black pepper
N'-Methyl-N'-nitroso-N-nitrosoguanidine (MNNG)	Pickled foods
N-Methyl-N-nitrosourea	Smoked, cured and grilled foods
Mineral oils	Rice, pasta, cereals, chocolate
Mirex	Contaminated food, especially root vegetables like carrots and potatoes
2-Napthalamine	Fumes of commercial sunflower, vegetable, and lard oil
Nickel	Fish, scallops, green leafy vegetables, oats, cocoa, coffee, tea, beans and legumes, canned foods; foods cooked in nickel vessels
Nitrates and nitrites	Processed meats such as ham, bacon, hot dogs, deli meat
Nitrofen (2,4-dichlorophenyl-p-nitrophenyl ether)	Pesticide contamination of food
1-Nitropyrene	Rice, vegetables, grilled foods
N-Nitrosodiethylamine	Processed foods and beverages such as cured meats, bacon, cheeses, whiskey, beer, water
N-Nitrosodimethylamine (NMDA)	Processed foods and beverages such as cured meats, bacon, and cheeses, whiskey, beer, and water
N-nitroso-N-methylurea	Nitrate-preserved food, meat, grains, and some vegetables
N-nitrosomethylvinylamine; N-nitrosomorpholine; N-nitrosonornicotine; N-nitrosopiperidine; N-nitrosopyrrolidine; and N-nitrososarcosine	Cured meats, primarily cooked bacon; beer; some cheeses; nonfat dry milk; some fish
Non-arsenical pesticides in food	Crop foods

Table 21 continued

Anticipated to be Human Carcinogens		
Effects on humans	IARC	NTP
Probable human carcinogen	2a	
Reasonably anticipated to be a human carcinogen		2a
Joint pain, developmental delay, learning disabilities, vomiting, abdominal pain, irritability, loss of appetite and weight loss, seizures, hearing loss,	2a	2a
Reasonably anticipated to be a human carcinogen		2a
Bladder cancer	1	
Photosensitivity, fatigue, nausea, dizziness, fatigue, probable human carcinogen	2a	
Reasonably anticipated to be a human carcinogen		2a
Gastric cancer, hepatocellular cancer, other GI cancers	2a	2a
Nausea, vomiting, headache, alkylates DNA, probable human carcinogen	2a	
Diarrhea, upset stomach, bowel damage, malnutrition, pneumonia if inhaled; untreated or mildly treated cause skin and scrotal cancer; possibly bladder, pancreatic, stomach, rectal, lung, sinonasal, and laryngeal cancer	1	1
Reasonably anticipated to be a human carcinogen		2a
Bladder cancer	1	1
Itching, rash, warm tender skin, dermatitis, blisters; lung and nasal cancer	1	1
Colon cancer, increase heart disease risk, blood vessel damage, stomach ache		
Reasonably anticipated to be a human carcinogen		2a
Probable human carcinogen	2a	2a
Headache, fever, nausea, jaundice, vomiting, abdominal cramps, hepatomegaly, dizziness, impaired liver, kidney and lung function; probable human carcinogen	2a	2a
Headache, fever, nausea, jaundice, vomiting, abdominal cramps, hepatomegaly, dizziness, impaired liver, kidney and lung function; probable human carcinogen	2a	2a
Reasonably anticipated to be a human carcinogen		2a
Reasonably anticipated to be a human carcinogen		2a
Probable human carcinogen	2a	

Table 21 continued

Substances in our Food Supply that are Known Carcinogens or Reasonably	
Carcinogen	**Found in these foods**
Ochratoxin A	Cereals and cereal products, coffee, cocoa, wine, beer, spices, dried fruits, grape juice, meat contaminated with this mycotoxin
Opisthorchis viverrine (Southeast Asian liver fluke)	Undercooked fish containing larvae
3,4,5,3',4'-Pentachlorobiphenyl (PCB-126)	Food preservatives, fungistat in packaging of citrus fruits, has been found in drinking water
2,3,4,7,8-Pentachloro-dibenzofuran	Seafood
Petroleum	Food colorings and additives
Phophorus-32, as phosphate	Chicken, turkey, pork, organ meats, seafood, dairy, sunflower and pumpkin seeds, nuts, whole grains
Polybrominated biphenyls (PBBs)	Oils and fats, fish and shellfish, meat and meat products, eggs
Polychlorinated biphenyls (PCBs)	Dairy, fish, shellfish, animal fat
Polycyclic aromatic hydrocarbons (PAH)	Shellfish (especially mussels and oysters); foods that are smoked or dried; grilled meat
Processed meat	Meat
Progesterone	Beans, broccoli, Brussels sprouts, nuts, pumpkin, spinach, whole grains, cauliflower, kale, pumpkin
Beta-Propiolactone	Sterilant for water, milk, and nutrient broth
Radon and radioactivity in foods	Water, bananas, Brazil nuts, beans, potatoes, carrots, red meat, avocados, beer, low sodium salt, peanut butter
Red meat	Chemicals such as heterocyclic amines, polycyclic aromatic hydrocarbons, N-nitroso compounds, trimethylamine N-oxide, antibiotics, hormones, dioxins, etc.
Safrole	Pumpkin pie, nutmeg, pepper, star anise, essential oils like sassafras
Salted fish, Chinese	N-nitroso compounds formed during production and steaming
Schistosoma haematobium infection	Consumption of contaminated water that contains parasite eggs
Selenium (elemental) and selenium salts	Contaminated drinking water and wastewater
Silica, as quartz or cristobalite	As silicone dioxide, an anti-caking agent; in liquids and beverages, an anti-foaming agent; green beans, bananas, leafy greens, brown rice, cereal, lentils, beer
Styrene and Styrene-7,8-oxide	Baked goods, frozen dairy products, candy, gelatin, pudding, fruits, and vegetables

Table 21 continued

Anticipated to be Human Carcinogens		
Effects on humans	**IARC**	**NTP**
Reasonably anticipated to be a human carcinogen		2a
Biliary infections, stones, and cancer, hepatotoxic, eosinophilia, fever, chills, itch, abdominal pain, malaise, liver cancer (cholangiocarcinoma)	1	
Toxic to liver, kidneys, nervous system, nausea, indigestion, numbness, disruption of DNA, carcinogenic	1	
Skin irritation, immunotoxicity, congenital problems, hematologic issues, behavioral changes, endocrine abnormalities, developmental defects, cancer	1	
Irritation to skin, eye, nausea, headache, dizziness, death; probable human carcinogen	2a	
Diarrhea, can negatively affect body's ability to use minerals like iron, calcium, magnesium, and zinc; cardiotoxicity; premature aging, lung cancer	1	
Neurotoxicity, weight loss, skin disorders, liver, kidney, thyroid and immunotoxicity; probable human carcinogen	2a	2a
Breast, prostate, testicular, ovarian, and uterine cancer	1	2a
Reasonably anticipated to be a human carcinogen		2a
Pancreatic, prostate, stomach and colorectal cancer, type 2 diabetes	1	
Reasonably anticipated to be a human carcinogen		2a
Reasonably anticipated to be a human carcinogen		2a
Cancers, genetic defects, premature aging; high levels of exposure associated with leukemias, breast, bladder, colon, liver, lung, esophagus, ovaries, multiple myeloma, and stomach cancers	1	1
Probable human carcinogen	2a	
Reasonably anticipated to be a human carcinogen		2a
Cancer of nasopharynx and stomach	1	
Fever, abdominal pain, bloody diarrhea or stools, cough, fatigue, headache, rash and body aches; bladder cancer	1	
Reasonably anticipated to be a human carcinogen		2a
Upset stomach; lung cancer, silicosis, kidney disease, and COPD	1	1
Probable human carcinogen	2a	2a

Table 21 continued

Substances in our Food Supply that are Known Carcinogens or Reasonably	
Carcinogen	**Found in these foods**
Tetrabromobisphenol A (TBBPA)	Fish and shellfish, eggs
3,3',4,4'-Tetrachloroazobenzene (TCAB)	Residue on crop foods (used as pesticide)
2,3,7,8-Tetrachlorodibenzo-para-dioxin (TCDD); dioxin	Animal fats, meat, dairy, fish and shellfish, poultry, eggs
Tetrachloroethylene (perchloroethylene)	Found as contaminant in foods
Tetrafluoroethylene	Teflon surface on cooking pans
Thiourea	Brassica vegetables
Toluene diisocyanate (TDI)	Fatty foods such as meat, poultry, seafood, milk, egg, and their products
Toxaphene	Shellfish and fish
Trichloroethylene	Water
2,4,6-Trichlorophenol	Pesticide contaminated food and water
1,2,3-Trichloropropane	Water
Urethane	Fermented food products and alcoholic beverages including soy sauce, kimchi, and breads, along with wine and sake
Very hot beverages	Tea, coffee, other hot drinks
Vinyl bromide	Food, from bromide containing fumigants used in horticulture
Vinyl chloride	Plastic bottles and containers for food, water, and beverages
Vinyl fluoride	Food

Adapted from following resources:
US Department of Health and Human Services. 15th report on carcinogens. National Toxicology Program website. Published December 21, 2021. Accessed July 8, 2022. https://ntp.niehs.nih.gov/whatwestudy/assessments/cancer/roc/index.html.
International Agency for Research on Cancer (IARC). Agents classified by the IARC monographs, Volumes 1–132. 2022. IARC website. Updated August 12, 2022. Accessed July 8, 2022. https://monographs.iarc.who.int/agents-classified-by-the-iarc/.
International Agency for Research on Cancer (IARC). Preamble to the IARC monographs. IARC website. Updated June 4, 2019. Accessed July 8, 2022. Accessed at https://monographs.iarc.fr/preamble-to-the-iarc-monographs/.

Table 21 continued

Anticipated to be Human Carcinogens

Effects on humans	IARC	NTP
Probable human carcinogen	2a	
Probable human carcinogen	2a	
Chloracne, a skin condition, skin rashes, excess body hair, skin discoloration; breast cancer	1	1
Vinyl chloride disease (Raynaud's phenomenon (blanching, numbness, and discomfort of the fingers upon exposure to cold), degeneration of the fingertip bones (acroosteolysis), joint and muscle pain, hepatotoxicity; probable human carcinogen	2a	2a
Stable when used for cooking and not ingested; flu-like symptoms, fever, chills, headache, chest pain; probable human carcinogen	2a	2a
Reasonably anticipated to be a human carcinogen		2a
Reasonably anticipated to be a human carcinogen		2a
Reasonably anticipated to be a human carcinogen		2a
Flushing, liver dysfunction, CNS depression, kidney cancer, Hodgkins lymphoma, possibly liver cancer	1	1
Reasonably anticipated to be a human carcinogen		2a
Probable human carcinogen	2a	2a
Probable human carcinogen		2a
Esophageal cancer	2a	
Probable human carcinogen; thought to have same effects as vinyl chloride	2a	2a
CNS toxicity, liver cancer (hepatic angiosarcoma), brain and lung cancer, lymphoma, and leukemia	1	1
Probable human carcinogen; thought to have same effects as vinyl chloride	2a	2a

Charts of Food-Related Reactions

FOOD-INDUCED ALLERGIC REACTIONS

Allergic reactions involve one or more body systems. Symptoms of a mild allergic reaction affect one organ system. For example, hay fever affects the upper respiratory system. In contrast, a severe allergic reaction involves two or more body systems.

These pages contain descriptions of three types of food-induced allergic reactions that range from mild to severe and from acute to chronic.

SUDDEN, MILD SYMPTOMS
FOOD ALLERGY
(FOOD HYPERSENSITIVITY)

SYMPTOMS
NOSE—Itchy, runny nose, sneezing, coughing
THROAT—Itchy
MOUTH—Tingling, itchy after eating
SKIN—Few hives, mild itch, eczema, rash
GUT—Headache, nausea, vomiting, diarrhea

CAUSE
Your immune system's response to an allergic trigger.

ACTION STEPS
1. Give antihistamines if prescribed by doctor.
2. Identify the offending food and avoid it.

WHEN TO VISIT AN ALLERGIST
If you suspect an allergy, to validate the allergy, and for advice on treatment and prognosis.

If needed, your allergist will test you to determine the amount of the food trigger/allergen you can safely consume.

SUDDEN, SEVERE SYMPTOMS
SEVERE FOOD ALLERGY ANAPHYLAXIS

SYMPTOMS

Respiratory problems that may be life-threatening.

LUNGS–Shortness of breath, wheezing, repetitive cough

MOUTH–Significant swelling of tongue and/or lips

THROAT–Tight, hoarse, trouble breathing, swallowing

HEART– Pale, blue skin, weak pulse, dizzy

SKIN–Many hives, widespread redness

GUT–Repetitive vomiting, severe diarrhea

MOOD–Feeling something bad is about to happen

COMBINATION–Both severe and mild symptoms affecting different parts of body.

CAUSE

Your immune system's response to an allergic trigger.

ACTION STEPS

Use your Anaphylaxis Action Plan.

If you do not have one, follow these steps:

1. INJECT epinephrine.
2. CALL 911 for an ambulance.
3. Monitor symptoms, as a second anaphylactic attack can occur. You can safely give two injections of epinephrine.
4. DO NOT depend on antihistamines or inhalers to treat severe symptoms.

WHEN TO VISIT AN ALLERGIST

See your allergist immediately.

DELAYED SYMPTOMS IN INFANTS AND CHILDREN

Non-IgE MEDIATED FOOD ALLERGY

SYMPTOMS

Intestinal symptoms signaling a delayed allergic reaction occur within minutes to hours after child ingests food allergen.

AP–Food Protein-Induced Allergic Proctocolitis (milk/soy)–Blood and mucus in stool; gas and abdominal pain.

FPE–Food Protein-Induced Enteropathy Refractory diarrhea, vomiting, malabsorption; failure to thrive.

FPIES–Food Protein-Induced Enterocolitis Syndrome (milk/soy)–Significant vomiting, diarrhea, dehydration; failure to thrive.

Heiner's Syndrome–Chronic respiratory issues, anemia, fever; failure to thrive.

CAUSE

Cells attack the intestinal walls.

ACTION STEPS

1. Treat symptoms of dehydration.
2. Identify the offending food and avoid it.

WHEN TO VISIT AN ALLERGIST

See your allergist immediately.

FOOD INDUCED NON-ALLERGIC REACTIONS

Non-allergic reactions such as food intolerance generally affect just one primary body system and can also be caused by inadequate gut enzymes, exposure to poison/toxic materials, or a pollen allergy.

For example, lactose intolerance affects the gastrointestinal system with symptoms of bloating, nausea, etc.

These pages contain descriptions of three types of food-induced reactions that have symptoms that look like allergies, but are not.

CHRONIC, MILD SYMPTOMS
OR PATTERN OF SYMPTOMS

FOOD INTOLERANCE

SYMPTOMS
NOSE–Itchy, runny nose, sneezing
MOUTH–Tingling, itchy
JOINTS–Pain, ache
SKIN–Chronic rash and discomfort
GUT–Pain, bloating, diarrhea, constipation, nausea, IBS

CAUSE
Not an allergy, but the body responds because it doesn't produce the enzymes necessary to break down the proteins in specific foods or is unable to absorb specific nutrients such as the lactose in cow's milk or fat.

ACTION
1. Identify the food(s) that cause your symptoms.
2. Read FODMAP and other resources to learn about major allergens you may not tolerate. See Chapter 20, Figure 54.

WHEN TO SEE AN ALLERGIST
An allergist can help you determine the amount of the sensitizing food you can safely consume without symptoms. If symptoms become severe, see an allergist. For more details, see Chapter 20.

ACUTE or CHRONIC DELAYED SYMPTOMS

FOOD TOXICITY

SYMPTOMS

Symptoms appear in the body system exposed to the toxin. Severity of symptoms is dose-dependent.
LUNGS—Inhalation of toxin can damage the lungs, cause lung cancer, e.g. asbestos.
SKIN—Skin contact with the toxin may cause neurological symptoms like tingling fingertips.
GUT—Ingestion of toxin may overload the filtering capabilities of the kidneys and liver over time.

CAUSE

Literally a result of ingesting something poisonous, such as pesticides from food and Teflon from cooking pans. May take years for body to reflect toxic poisoning or, in case of acute poisoning, may be immediate.

Food Toxicity can also be caused by food poisoning, an acute reaction to eating food contaminated with bacteria, viruses, or parasites.

ACTION
1. Identify the cause and avoid it.
2. Prevention is key: Store food properly and eat only fresh food that is properly sourced.

WHEN TO SEE A DOCTOR

If symptoms are mild, see your primary care Doctor. For acute poisoning, go to the Emergency Dept. For more details, see Chapter 21.

SUDDEN, MILD SYMPTOMS AFTER EATING SPECIFIC RAW FRUITS AND VEGETABLES

ORAL ALLERGY SYNDROME

SYMPTOMS
LIPS, MOUTH, TONGUE—Tingling, itchy

CAUSE

People with pollen allergies may react to fruits and vegetables that have similar proteins to their pollen allergen. Reaction may be limited to high-pollen seasons for some.

ACTION
1. Take antihistamines.
2. Review list of foods and their pollen counterparts for related foods to avoid. See Chapter 12, Figure 33.
3. Avoid raw forms of the fruits and vegetables to which you react. Try other forms, such as sautéed vegetables, cooked fruit sauces, baked apples. Also try eating the food after heating, peeling, or dipping in lemon juice.

WHEN TO SEE AN ALLERGIST

See an Allergist to rule out other causes and confirm diagnosis. Also, if there is escalation of symptoms or unexpected symptoms. See Chapter 12.

ACUTE OR CHRONIC REACTIONS ASSOCIATED WITH FOOD

These pages contain descriptions of three additional types of non-allergic reactions that are associated with food, but caused by other substances or conditions.

These conditions present with acute to chronic and mild to severe symptoms (or a pattern of symptoms) and are less likely to occur in children.

ACUTE or CHRONIC, MILD to SEVERE SYMPTOMS OR PATTERN OF SYMPTOMS

FOOD INTOLERANCE ASSOCIATED WITH MEDICATION

SYMPTOMS
Many and varied, dependent on the drug. Can increase or decrease the side effects or activity of the original medication; can alter functioning or damage an organ; can cause death.

CAUSE
Increase or decrease specific liver enzymes; increase or decrease albumin; increase or decrease the blood concentration, absorption, elimination, bioavailability, or activity of a medication.

ACTION
1. Identify the medication(s) that cause your symptoms and reduce or discontinue that medication. Also, avoid the food that causes the interaction.
2. See Tables 15 and 16, Food-Drug Interactions in Chapter 21.

WHEN TO SEE A DOCTOR
If symptoms are mild, see your Primary Care Doctor.

ACUTE or CHRONIC, MILD to SEVERE
SYMPTOMS OR PATTERN OF SYMPTOMS

FOOD INTOLERANCE ASSOCIATED WITH DISEASE

SYMPTOMS
NOSE–Itchy, runny nose, sneezing
MOUTH–Tingling, itchy
JOINTS–Pain, ache
SKIN–Chronic rash, discomfort
GUT–pain, bloating, diarrhea, constipation, nausea

CAUSE
Not an allergy
Immune deficiencies
Rosacea, acne
Headache (and/or migraine)
Depression, mental health
Autism
Obesity and diabetes

ACTION
1. Identify the food(s) that cause your symptoms.
2. Determine the amount of the sensitizing food you can safely consume without symptoms.
3. Learn more about major food allergens you or your child may not tolerate. See Chapter 7.

WHEN TO VISIT AN ALLERGIST
If you suspect an allergy, to validate the allergy, and for advice on treatment and prognosis.
If symptoms become severe, visit an allergist.

WHEN TO SEE A DOCTOR
If symptoms are mild, see your Primary Care Doctor.

ACUTE or CHRONIC, MILD to SEVERE
SYMPTOMS OR PATTERN OF SYMPTOMS

FOOD AVERSION

SYMPTOMS
Many and varied, may mimic a known disease state, most commonly nausea, vomiting, and abdominal pain.

CAUSE
Traumatic experience at a time proximate to consuming a specific food; or due to high sensitivity due to food.

ACTION
Be assured that food aversion is a genuine medical concern and help is available.

WHEN TO SEE A DOCTOR
If symptoms are mild, see your Primary Care Doctor.

WHEN TO VISIT AN ALLERGIST
If you suspect an allergy; to validate or rule out an allergy.

Helpful Resources for Allergic Patients and Their Families

Organization	Website
Governmental Health Resources (United States)	
Centers for Disease Control	www.cdc.gov
Environmental Protection Agency	https://www.epa.gov
Food and Drug Administration	http://www.fda.gov/
World Health Organization (International)	https://www.who.int
National Institutes of Health (United States)	
Consumer Product Information Database	https://www.whatsinproducts.com/
National Heart, Lung, and Blood Institute - Asthma Guidelines	http://www.nhlbi.nih.gov/guidelines/asthma/asthgdln.htm
National Institute of Diabetes, Digestive & Kidney Diseases	http://www2.niddk.nih.gov/
National Institute of Neurologic Diseases & Stroke	https://www.ninds.nih.gov
National Library of Medicine	https://medlineplus.gov
National Toxicology Program	https://ntp.niehs.nih.gov
Allergy, Intolerance, Toxicity Resources	
American Academy of Allergy, Asthma & Immunology	https://aaaai.org
American Board of Allergy and Immunology	https://abai.org
American College of Allergy, Asthma & Immunology	https://acaai.org
Cancer Resources	
Agency for Toxic Substances and Disease Registry (CDC)	https://www.atsdr.cdc.gov/
American Cancer Society	http://www.cancer.org/Research/CancerFactsFigures/index
International Agency for Research on Cancer (WHO)	https://monographs.iarc.who.int/

National Cancer Institute of the NIH	https://www.cancer.gov/
Oncolink – information resources about cancer	https://www.oncolink.org
Celiac Disease	
Patient advocacy and research-driven organization	https://www.beyondceliac.org/celiac-disease/
Source for at-home celiac testing	https://www.imaware.health/at-home-blood-test/celiac-disease-screening
Clinical Trial Resources	
United States	http://www.clinicaltrials.gov
European Union	https://www.clinicaltrialsregister.eu/
National Organization of Rare Diseases Resource of Clinical Trials	https://rarediseases.org/for-patients-and-families/information-resources/info-clinical-trials-and-research-studies/
Genetic and Rare Diseases (GARD) Information Center	http://rarediseases.info.nih.gov/GARD/
Contact Allergy and Dermatology	
Contact allergen database	http://contactallergy.com/
Contact Dermatitis Institute Allergen Database	https://www.contactdermatitisinstitute.com/database.php
New Zealand Dermatologic Society	https://dermnetnz.org/
SkinSAFE mobile application	https://www.skinsafeproducts.com/apps
Eosinophilic Diseases	
American Partnership for Eosinophilic Diseases (APFED)	https://apfed.org/
Campaign Urging Research for Eosinophilic Disease (CURED)	http://www.curedfoundation.org
Food Allergy Resources	
Food Allergy Research & Education	https://foodallergy.org
Food Allergy Research & Resource Program	https://farrp.unl.edu/

| Food Allergen Labeling and Consumer Protection Act | http://www.fda.gov/food/foodsafety/foodallergies |
| InformAll Allergenic Food Database | http://research.bmh.manchester.ac.uk/informall/allergenic-foods/ |

Headache, Migraine Resources

American Migraine Foundation	https://www.achenet.org
Association of Migraine Disorders	https://www.migrainedisorders.org
National Headache Foundation	https://www.headaches.org

Miscellaneous Resources

Chemicals sold by country	https://www.chemicalbook.com
Chemical information database	https://pubchem.ncbi.nlm.nih.gov/
Food safety	https://www.foodwatch.org/en/foodwatch-international/
Information for common health and wellness topics	https://www.healthline.com/
Pesticide residue reports and data (FDA)	https://www.fda.gov/food/pesticides/pesticide-residue-monitoring-program-reports-and-data
Watchdog group uncovering industrial corruption	https://www.sourcewatch.org/index.php?title=SourceWatch

Glossary

<u>Allergist-Immunologist (commonly referred to as an allergist)</u>: A physician who is specially trained to diagnose, treat, and manage allergies, asthma, and immunologic disorders, including primary immunodeficiency disorders. In the United States, becoming an allergist-immunologist requires at least an additional nine years of training beyond a bachelor's degree.

After completing medical school and graduating with a medical degree, physicians undergo three years of training in Internal Medicine or Pediatrics, then pass the exam of either the American Board of Internal Medicine (ABIM) or the American Board of Pediatrics (ABP). Following that, becoming an allergist-immunologist requires at least two additional years of study, called a fellowship, in an Allergy-Immunology training program. A board-certified allergist-immunologist passes exams composed by the American Board of Allergy & Immunology (ABAI) on a regular basis throughout their career.

<u>Allergy</u>: Overreaction of the body to a normally harmless substance (pollen, dog dander, etc.). This reaction is caused by the immune system, the body system that defends us from foreign invaders. Because the body seems to get confused about the threat level of the foreign substance, it can respond vigorously and sometimes in a life-threatening manner (see <u>anaphylaxis</u>). Also known as a <u>hypersensitivity reaction</u>.

<u>Acne</u>: A skin condition in which the hair follicles become filled with skin cells and oil and can become plugged, red, and cause painful bumps on the skin.

<u>Acquired angioedema</u>: A type of angioedema (see <u>angioedema</u>) caused by another chronic condition, characteristically an autoimmune disease or cancer.

<u>Allergic rhinitis</u> (also known as hay fever) includes symptoms such as nasal congestion, postnasal drip, rhinorrhea; itchy, red and runny eyes; and coughing and sneezing. It is a typical reaction to environmental allergens like pollen from grass, weeds, trees, ragweed, mold spores, and animal dander.

<u>Alpha-Gal allergy</u> is a severe and potentially life-threatening food allergy to a carbohydrate molecule (galactose-alpha-1,3-galactose) found in most mammalian or red meat. It is caused by a tick bite, which causes exposure to this protein.

Analgesic medications are pain medications and, in this book, the term specifically refers to opioids (hydrocodone, oxycodone) and nonsteroidal anti-inflammatory (NSAID) medications (naproxen, ibuprofen), as these cause the chemical mediators in the allergic cells to increase, making them more prone to causing a severe allergic reaction.

Anaphylaxis is a severe type of allergic reaction (see Chapter 6) distinguished from a mild or moderate allergic reaction by the sudden involvement of two or more organ systems, manifesting with a variety of symptoms, such as difficulty breathing, swelling of the tongue, swelling or tightness in the throat, wheezing, sudden persistent cough, abdominal pain, vomiting, and hypotension. It is potentially life-threatening and is the most extreme form of allergy or hypersensitivity.

Anaphylaxis Action Plan is a plan that contains step-by-step medical directions explaining how to respond to anaphylaxis. Your Anaphylaxis Action Plan is created for you by your child's allergist-immunologist.

Anaphylatoxins are mediators made and released by allergy cells during an allergic reaction. They cause lung constriction, swelling, blood vessel leakage, and other symptoms of allergy.

Angioedema is the swelling of the deeper layers of the skin, caused by a buildup of fluid. The symptoms of angioedema can affect any part of the body, but swelling usually affects the eyes, lips, genitals, hands, and feet. Many people with angioedema also experience urticaria (hives). There are many causes of angioedema: it can be inherited, a reaction to cancer or an autoimmune disease, or an allergy from a medication, food, environmental pollen, or contact with a substance.

Angiotensin-converting enzyme (ACE) inhibitors or Angiotensin receptor blockers (ARB) are medications typically used for blood pressure control and sometimes for kidney protection in diabetes. While excellent medications for these issues, events such as hives, cough, and swelling are side effects that are unanticipated. If any of these side effects happen, the medication should likely be discontinued, and a substitute found. These issues can happen at any time.

Antihistamine is a type of medication used to block the effects of histamine, one of the principal allergic chemicals released from the cells of allergy. Examples of antihistamines include diphenhydramine (Benadryl), cetirizine (Zyrtec), levocetirizine (Xyzal), loratadine (Claritin), and fexofenadine (Allegra).

Antileukotriene is a type of medication used to block leukotriene. The most common example is montelukast (Singulair).

Asthma is a serious chronic lung disease causing inflammation of the lungs characterized by intermittent or persistent symptoms of shortness of breath, wheezing, chest tightness, and/or cough. These symptoms worsen in the presence of specific triggers.

Asthma Action Plan is a plan that consists of step-by-step medical directions explaining how to respond to an asthma flare. The intent is to help you get your child's care started to prevent his/her asthma from getting worse and perhaps avoid use of the emergency room or urgent care. Your Asthma Action Plan is created for you by your child's allergist-immunologist.

Autism refers to a broad range of developmental conditions characterized by challenges in social skills, repetitive behaviors, fixation on fields of interest, nonverbal communication, and speech. According to the CDC, it affects 1 in 44 children in the United States.

Autoantibodies are directed against a specific part of your child's body, potentially allowing your child's immune system to attack their body. They are usually not a problem because the cells that make them are weeded out. If the cells get past the normal regulation, the antibodies are problematic if they function (turn something off that should be on; turn something on that should be off) or are effective at causing damage. Autoantibodies are thought to be the pathology behind most chronic idiopathic urticaria (hives), thyroid disease, rheumatoid arthritis, lupus, multiple sclerosis, and many other issues.

Autoimmunity is when the body attacks itself. This is characteristically caused by autoantibodies (see autoantibodies).

Atopic dermatitis (eczema) Atopic dermatitis is the most common type of eczema and appears as a red, itchy rash or dry, scaly plaques of skin. While it can develop at any age, it usually begins in infancy or young childhood.

Aversion is a term to describe a strong dislike that causes avoidance.

B cells, also known as basophils or "white cells," are cells of the immune system. They make antibodies or immunoglobulin, including Immunoglobulin E (IgE, the allergic flag), which flags certain cells for destruction, including foreign invaders such as allergens, bacteria, viruses, and parasites.

Basophils are one type of the cells in circulation in the body's immune system that defend it against foreign invaders such as allergens, bacteria, viruses, and parasites. See B cells.

Bradykinin is a peptide that promotes inflammation. It is released from immune cells and causes increased inflammation, regulation of blood pressure, blood vessel leakage, and pain.

Carcinogenic is a term that describes a substance that causes cancer.

C1 esterase inhibitor is a protein that decreases activity of C1 esterase, keeping its activity in check. Loss of control is seen when it is missing or decreased, such as in C1 esterase inhibitor deficiency, and this causes C1 esterase, part of the complement system, to act unchecked, causing swelling of tissues when the immune mediators are produced without its inhibitory effect, typically of the face and hands.

Celiac disease is a non-IgE-mediated gluten allergy or hypersensitivity. This food protein-induced small intestinal disease goes by multiple names, including gluten enteropathy, celiac sprue, sprue, and Celiac disease. Symptoms may include chronic diarrhea, rash, and signs of malabsorption in the part of the gut that absorbs iron, resulting in iron-deficiency anemia.

Contact dermatitis is a rash, swelling, and itch found at the area of skin contact with the allergen.

Cross-contamination occurs when an allergenic food is mixed with or touches a non-allergenic food, thereby making it unsafe for the highly allergic person to consume.

Cross-reactive foods are foods that an allergic person is more likely to react to because they have a common protein structure with the patient's allergenic food.

Cytokines are like hormones of the immune system that cause another cell or cells to respond in a specific way. They typically cause increased or decreased inflammation.

Delayed-type allergy is an allergy caused by cells that attack the body, causing injury. Because the cells take longer to activate and move to the area where they cause damage, these allergies are called delayed hypersensitivity reactions and are also known as Type IV allergies. This is one type of a non-IgE-mediated allergy.

Dermatitis herpetiformis is a skin rash consisting of intensely itchy clusters of blisters and is caused by deposition of immunoglobulin A (the immunoglobulin typically found in mucosal membranes) in the skin, triggering inflammation. It is the skin manifestation of celiac disease.

The Dietary Inflammatory Index (DII) is an index in which inflammatory points are assigned to foods that have a significant impact on health, obesity, and diabetes. The DII was calculated based on inflammatory parameters provoked by individual foods when consumed in isolation.

Epinephrine is the "fight or flight" hormone; it is also the antidote to anaphylaxis or severe allergy as it reverses many of the symptoms that would otherwise be life-threatening.

Eczema appears as a red, itchy rash or dry, scaly plaques of skin. While it can develop at any age, it usually begins in infancy or young childhood.

Elemental diet is a diet entirely dependent on a formula that has no proteins, but only amino acids, sugars, and essential fatty acids. It is designed to be as hypoallergenic as possible without complete avoidance of nutrition. It generally refers to baby formula.

Eosinophilic colitis (EC) is caused by infiltration, injury, and inflammation produced by eosinophils, a type of white blood cell in the large intestine. Symptoms include abdominal pain, nausea, vomiting, diarrhea (which may be bloody), weight loss, anemia, fatigue, and malnutrition.

Eosinophilic esophagitis (EoE) is a chronic immunologic condition that causes inflammation of the esophagus, the tube that moves food between the mouth and stomach. EoE is named after the eosinophils, one type of white blood cell, found in higher than normal numbers in damaged areas of the esophagus.

Eosinophilic gastroenteritis is a rare disorder that can involve any portion of the gastrointestinal tract but tends to cause eosinophilic invasion in one or more layers of the walls of the stomach and/or intestine.

Eosinophils are a disease-fighting white blood cell that defends the body against foreign invaders such as allergens, bacteria, viruses, and parasites.

Extensively hydrolyzed infant formula is a formula that has been broken down into small pieces, known as peptides, and in doing so, it makes the formula less able to cause an allergic reaction, such as whole milk infant formula, as the allergy-causing pieces are broken down in the process.

FODMAPs (Fermentable Oligosaccharides, D-saccharides, Monosaccharides and Polyols) are difficult to digest carbohydrates that cause digestive distress.

Food intolerance presents as uncomfortable symptoms after eating specific foods. The typical symptom pattern is loose stools to diarrhea, abdominal pain, bloating and distention, and altered motility that occurs shortly after eating specific foods.

Food Oral Challenge is a technique in which small doses of food are fed to someone and then slowly increased under observation to validate or rule out a food as an allergy for that patient.

Food Oral Immunotherapy (FOIT) is the highly-controlled process of decreasing the allergic response and increasing tolerance of the immune system to food. This is done by the allergist-immunologist, who feeds the food beginning at levels below the allergic threshold and increasing slowly until a maintenance dose is achieved. It is used in patients with an anaphylactic response to the food. FOIT is typically performed with the intent to make the anaphylaxis survivable or not occur at all and, in some cases, free eating can be achieved.

Food protein-induced enterocolitis syndrome (FPIES) is a food allergy that presents as significant, often projectile and repetitive vomiting, diarrhea, dehydration, lethargy, and failure to thrive. It can also cause metabolic derangements, hypotension, and hypothermia.

Food protein-induced allergic proctocolitis (AP) is a food allergy that typically presents as blood-streaked, highly mucous stools as well as an increase in gas.

Food Protein-Induced Enteropathy (FPE) is a food allergy that begins within the first nine months of a child's life, usually starting when soy or cow's milk formula is introduced. Other triggers may present later when other foods are incorporated into the diet. FPE presents as refractory diarrhea, vomiting, malabsorption, and abdominal distention, as well as failure to thrive and abdominal pain, especially on defecation.

Food Protein-Induced Enteropathy (FPE) begins within the first nine months, usually starting when soy or cow's milk formula is introduced and presents with symptoms of refractory diarrhea, vomiting, malabsorption, and abdominal distention, as well as failure to thrive.

Food & Drug Administration (FDA)-approved medication refers to a medication approved for a specific condition by the Center for Drug Evaluation and Research. A medication not approved by the FDA can be used for a specific condition at the discretion of a physician. Physicians may do this if they are aware that a medication is about to be approved for that condition or if they are aware that it is effective clinically for that condition but that the manufacturer has not submitted that medication to the FDA for use in that condition, perhaps due to the extreme expense of this process. It currently costs approximately $2-$3 billion to develop and research a drug for a specific disease process.

Heiner's Syndrome (pulmonary hemosiderosis) is a reaction primarily triggered by cow's milk in infancy. Symptoms include chronic, recurrent respiratory issues, anemia, recurrent fever, and hemoptysis (coughing up blood) with resulting wheezing, short-ness of breath, and visible pulmonary infiltrates on chest X-ray. Some children experience failure to gain weight and failure to thrive.

Histamine is a chemical released from allergic cells that causes symptoms of allergy, including constriction of muscles, making breathing difficult, dilation of blood vessels, causing flushing and low blood pressure as well as runny nose, itching, red runny eyes, nasal congestion, and other symptoms that can range from hay fever-like symptoms to anaphylaxis.

Hives (or urticaria) is a mosquito-bite-like rash consisting of a wheal (where the rash is swollen and red in the center) and flare (where there is a surrounding redness that is not swollen) that is very itchy and sometimes painful. There are many causes of hives, including allergy and autoimmunity, in the case of chronic idiopathic urticaria.

IgE-mediated allergy - see Immediate-type allergy.

Immediate-type allergy is an allergy caused by the interaction of allergic cells with Immunoglobulin E (IgE) latched onto the allergic substance. This interaction causes the allergic cells to release histamine and chemicals of the allergic response. The symptoms of immediate-type allergy include shortness of breath, wheezing, hoarse-ness, nausea, abdominal pain, diarrhea, vomiting, hives, itching, flushing, low blood pressure, cramping and loss of bladder and bowel control, angioedema, asthma, and anaphylaxis, and can lead to loss of consciousness and death. This is called immediate-type allergy because it happens rapidly after exposure to an allergic substance and is also known as Type I allergy or IgE-mediated allergy.

Immune system is the body system that defends us against viruses, bacteria, fungi, and other pathogens, targeting and destroying them in an attempt to prevent harm from the pathogens. This system regulates inflammation. It is the system that is dysfunctional in autoimmune disease and immunodeficiency.

Immunodeficiency is a condition caused by a defect in the immune system, the body system that defends against foreign invaders and cancer, resulting in increased infections from viruses, bacteria, fungi, as well as increased risk of cancers. Some immunodeficiency diseases are accompanied by a tendency for autoimmunity as well.

Immunoglobulin E (Ig E) is the allergic antibody that flags allergens and pathogens to alert the immune system, the body's defense system, to their presence so that they may be eliminated.

Immunoglobulin IgG is an antibody that flags intracellular viruses, bacteria, and fungi to alert the immune system, the body's defense system, to their presence so that they may be eliminated.

Inhaled corticosteroids (ICS) are inhaled medications used for asthma. They have an anti-inflammatory effect on the lungs, which is why they are used for asthma and other lung diseases. Inhaled corticosteroids take about four weeks to take effect, which is why they are appropriate for maintenance of asthma but not for a rescue medication.

Intolerance - see Food intolerance.

Immunotherapy is a method to decrease the allergenicity of a substance or substances for a specific patient by carefully exposing the patient's immune system to the allergen over time, thus building up its tolerance and reducing the patient's risk of allergic reaction. Commonly known as "allergy shots" when used to control the allergic response to environment allergens such as pollens to grasses, trees, weeds, ragweed, animal dander, and molds. There is also a type of immunotherapy, food oral immunotherapy (see FOIT), to help build up food tolerance.

Irritable Bowel Syndrome (IBS) is a condition associated with recurrent abdominal pain that lasts at least one day per week and is present for at least three months during which time two or more of the following symptoms are present: the pain is associated with stooling, there is a change in stool frequency with the pain, or there is a change in stool form with the pain. IBS can be constipation-predominant, diarrhea-predominant, or a combination of the two, which is known as mixed.

Leukotrienes are a group of chemicals released by white blood cells that can regulate inflammation and allergic reactions.

Leukotriene antagonist (LTA) inhibits the effects of leukotrienes and therefore helps control allergic reactions and inflammation.

Leukotriene receptor antagonist (LTRA) prevents the effects of leukotrienes on the leukotriene receptors and therefore helps control allergic reactions and inflammation.

Long-acting beta agonists (LABA) are medications that relax the lungs and smooth muscle in the airways, causing easier breathing, and whose effects last about 12 hours.

Long-acting muscarinic agonists (LAMA) are medications that open lung airways, resulting in easier breathing, and whose effects last about 12 hours.

Mast cells are the cells of the immune system that play a pivotal role in allergic disease as well as in fighting certain infections. They are the "master allergic cells" and are located under the top layer of skin, around the blood vessels, and around the vital organs. They release histamines as well as other chemical mediators.

<u>Malabsorption</u> is a digestive disorder in which nutrients are not effectively absorbed.

<u>Metabolic</u> is a term referring to metabolism or the chemical processes that are necessary for life.

<u>Microbes</u> are small organisms such as bacteria, viruses, protozoa, or fungi. In this book, microbes can be beneficial (like in a healthy microbiome) or problematic (when they are pathogens).

<u>Microbiome</u> is a term referring to a group of microbes (bacteria, fungi, viruses) that live on or within the body. It is now understood that they all produce signals. Those that aid us in a metabolic task are regarded as "good" and those that contribute to disease or inhibit our metabolic tasks are regarded as "bad." The skin, gut, lungs, and sinuses are examples of areas of the body with a microbiome and the microbes of those areas "talk" to each other.

<u>Migraine</u> is a type of headache of varying intensity and duration characterized by pulsing, pounding, or throbbing, and it is often accompanied by nausea and vomiting as well as sensitivity to light and/or sound. It may be preceded by a warning that the migraine is about to occur, known as an aura, which is usually a visual disturbance, but can also be a sensory, auditory, or motor disturbance. Migraines can be disabling.

<u>Non-Ig E mediated allergy</u> - see <u>Delayed-type allergy</u>.

<u>Non-steroidal anti-inflammatory drugs (NSAIDs)</u> are drugs like naproxen, ibuprofen, and aspirin that decrease inflammation, pain, and fever. They do so by altering the inflammatory pathways.

<u>Obesity</u> is a state of having excess adipose tissue, defined as a body mass index (BMI) of 25 or more, which is considered a risk factor for many diseases and is now recognized as a state of increased inflammation.

<u>Oral allergy syndrome</u> is a mild form of allergy that occurs upon contact of the mouth and throat with certain raw fruits or vegetables. Oral allergy syndrome causes itching and swelling of the mouth, face, lips, tongue, and throat.

<u>Pathogens</u> are microbes such as bacteria, viruses, protozoans, or fungi that cause disease or are otherwise problematic to health.

<u>Patch testing</u> is a method of skin testing that involves prolonged contact of the skin with various substances for the purpose of determining delayed-type allergies that cause contact dermatitis and other Type IV (or delayed-type) allergies.

<u>Probiotics</u> are a mixture of bacteria and/or yeast that are designed to be consumed

and replete the gastrointestinal microbiome with "good" microbes and dilute the "bad" microbes.

Processing is any operation by which food is prepared for consumption.

Ragweed is a weed that is prevalent throughout the United States that generates pollen in spring and/or fall, depending on the area of the county. Ragweed causes symptoms of allergic rhinitis such as nasal congestion, postnasal drip, runny nose, and itchy, red, runny eyes.

Rosacea is a skin disease that can cause flushing, acne, redness, and even pain of the face. The nose may become bulbous and even disfigured. The blood vessels become enlarged and are visibly close to the skin surface.

Skin scratch (or prick) testing is the process by which immediate (or IgE-mediated) allergies to many substances can be identified. Scratching introduces the potential allergies to the allergic cells underneath the skin. If the substance is an allergen, the allergic cells release histamine, causing leakage of the blood vessels under the skin and dilation of the blood vessels under the skin, or a controlled hive, in that area. If the substance is not an allergen, no histamine is released and therefore no hive occurs.

Steroids (or corticosteroids) are a class of drug that are rapidly anti-inflammatory but have many side effects.

T cells are cells that act like the generals of the immune system, rallying it against foreign invaders such as bacteria, viruses, and fungi, tumors, and injuries. T cells orchestrate the immune response, possess a memory, and prevent attacks against entities the body needs or that are part of it.

Toxins are substances that are poisonous and can cause disease at relatively low levels in the body.

References

Agana M, Frueh J, Kamboj M, et al. Common metabolic disorder (inborn errors of metabolism) concerns in primary care practice. *Ann Transl Med*. 2018;6(24):469. doi: 10.21037/atm.2018.12.34. PMID: 30740400; PMCID: PMC6331353.

American Academy of Asthma, Allergy & Immunology (AAAAI). Eosinophilic esophagitis. AAAAI website. Updated February 24, 2020. Accessed December 6, 2021. https://www.aaaai.org/Conditions-Treatments/related-conditions/eosinophilic-esophagitis

American Academy of Asthma, Allergy & Immunology (AAAAI). Oral allergy syndrome (OAS). AAAAI website. Updated September 8, 2020. Accessed December 6, 2021. https://www.aaaai.org/Tools-for-the-Public/Conditions-Library/Allergies/Oral-allergy-syndrome-(OAS)

American Academy of Asthma, Allergy & Immunology (AAAAI). Alpha gal and red meat allergy. AAAAI website. Updated April 25, 2019. Accessed December 6, 2021. https://www.aaaai.org/tools-for-the-public/conditions-library/allergies/alpha-gal-and-red-meat-allergy

American Academy of Dermatology. Acne Resource Center American Academy of Dermatology website. Accessed December 8, 2021. https://www.aad.org/public/diseases/acne.

American Cancer Society. Cancer facts and figures 2010. American Cancer Society website. Accessed December 9, 2021. https://www.cancer.org/research/cancer-facts-statistics/all-cancer-facts-figures/cancer-facts-figures-2010.html

American College of Allergy, Asthma & Immunology (ACAAI). Eosinophilic Esophagitis. Updated May 23, 2022. Accessed September 12, 2022. https://acaai.org/allergies/allergic-conditions/eosinophilic-esophagitis/

American Lung Association, Epidemiology and Statistics Unit. Trends in asthma morbidity and mortality. American Lung Association website. Published 2012. Accessed December 7, 2021: https://www.lung.org/research/trends-in-lung-disease/asthma-trends-brief/trends-and-burden

Banerji A, Rudders SA, Corel B, et al. Predictors of hospital admission for food-related allergic reactions that present to the emergency department. *Ann Allergy Asthma Immunol*. 2011;106(1):42-8. doi: 10.1016/j.anai.2010.10.011. PMID: 21195944; PMCID: PMC3538809.

Barman, Malin. (2015). Long chain polyunsaturated fatty acids in serum phospholipids - relation to genetic polymorphisms, diet and allergy development in children.

Barnett SB, Nurmagambetov TA. Costs of asthma in the United States: 2002-2007. *J Allergy Clin Immunol*. 2011;127(1):145-52. doi: 10.1016/j.jaci.2010.10.020. PMID: 21211649.

Beyond Celiac. Celiac Disease Treatment. Beyond Celiac website. Accessed December 15, 2021. https://www.beyondceliac.org/celiac-disease/treatment.

Beyond Celiac. What is celiac disease? Beyond Celiac website. Accessed December 15, 2021. https://www.beyondceliac.org/celiac-disease

Biagini Myers JM, Khurana Hershey GK. Eczema in early life: genetics, the skin barrier, and lessons learned from birth cohort studies. *J Pediatr*. 2010;157(5):704-14. doi: 10.1016/j.jpeds.2010.07.009. Epub 2010 Aug 24. PMID: 20739029; PMCID: PMC2957505.

Bonilla, FA, Khan, DA MD, Ballas, ZK, et al. Joint Task Force on Practice Parameters, representing the American Academy of Allergy, Asthma & Immunology; the American College of Allergy, Asthma & Immunology; and the Joint Council of Allergy, Asthma & Immunology. Practice parameter for the diagnosis and management of primary immunodeficiency. *J Allergy Clin Immunol*. 2015;136(5):1186-205.e1-78. doi: 10.1016/j.jaci.2015.04.049. Epub 2015 Sep 12. PMID: 26371839.

Bork K, Staubach-Renz P, Hardt J. Angioedema due to acquired C1-inhibitor deficiency: spectrum and treatment with C1-inhibitor concentrate. *Orphanet J Rare Dis*. 2019;14(1):65. doi: 10.1186/s13023-019-1043-3. PMID: 30866985; PMCID: PMC6417199.

Boyce JA, Assa'ad A, Burks AW, et al.; NIAID-Sponsored Expert Panel. Guidelines for the diagnosis and management of food allergy in the United States: Summary of the NIAID-sponsored expert panel report. *J Allergy Clin Immunol*. 2010;126(6):1105-18. doi: 10.1016/j.jaci.2010.10.008. PMID: 21134568; PMCID: PMC4241958.

Bulnes S, Murueta-Goyena A, Lafuente JV. Differential exposure to N-ethyl N-nitrosourea during pregnancy is relevant to the induction of glioma and PNSTs in the brain. *Neurotoxicol Teratol*. 2021;86:106998. doi: 10.1016/j.ntt.2021.106998. Epub 2021 May 26. PMID: 34048896.

Bushra R, Aslam N, Khan AY. Food-drug interactions. *Oman Med J*. 2011;26(2):77-83. doi: 10.5001/omj.2011.21. PMID: 22043389; PMCID: PMC3191675.

Caminero A, Meisel M, Jabri B, Verdu EF. Mechanisms by which gut microorganisms influence food sensitivities. *Nat Rev Gastroenterol Hepatol*. 2019;16(1):7-18. doi: 10.1038/s41575-018-0064-z. PMID: 30214038; PMCID: PMC6767923.

Castro-Rodriguez JA, Forno E, Rodriguez-Martinez CE, Celedón JC. Risk and protective factors for childhood asthma: what is the evidence? *J Allergy Clin Immunol Pract*. 2016;4(6):1111-1122. doi: 10.1016/j.jaip.2016.05.003. Epub 2016 Jun 8. PMID: 27286779; PMCID: PMC5107168.

Castro-Rodríguez JA, Holberg CJ, Wright AL, Martinez FD. A clinical index to define risk of asthma in young children with recurrent wheezing. *Am J Respir Crit Care Med*. 2000;162(4 Pt 1):1403-6. doi: 10.1164/ajrccm.162.4.9912111. PMID: 11029352.

Centers for Disease Control; Agency for Toxic Substances and Disease Registry (ATSDR). ATSDR website. Accessed December 6-9, 2021. https://www.atsdr.cdc.gov/

Centers for Disease Control. Autism Spectrum Disorder. Diagnostic criteria. Updated November 2, 2022. Accessed December 2, 2022. https://www.cdc.gov/ncbddd/autism/hcp-dsm.html

Centers for Disease Control. Autism Spectrum Disorder. Signs and symptoms of autism spectrum disorder. Updated March 28, 2022. Accessed September 12, 2022. https://www.cdc.gov/ncbddd/autism/signs.html

Centers for Disease Control. How to prevent food poisoning. Centers for Disease Control Food Safety website. Updated April 15, 2022. Accessed August 26, 2022. https://www.cdc.gov/foodsafety/prevention.html

Centers for Disease Control. Morbidity and mortality weekly report. Centers for Disease Control website. Updated weekly. Accessed August 25, 2022. https://www.cdc.gov/mmwr

Centers for Disease Control. Most recent national asthma data. Updated May 25, 2022. Accessed December 6, 2021. https://www.cdc.gov/asthma/most_recent_national_asthma_data.htm

Centers for Disease Control. Flu vaccine and people with egg allergies. Centers for Disease Control website. Updated August 25, 2022. Accessed December 18, 2022. https://www.cdc.gov/flu/prevent/egg-allergies.htm

Centers for Disease Control; National Center for Emerging and Zoonotic Infectious Diseases (NCEZID), Division of Foodborne, Waterborne, and Environmental Diseases (DFWED); Foodborne germs and illness. Centers for Disease Control and Prevention website. Updated March 18, 2020. Accessed December 7, 2021. https://www.cdc.gov/foodsafety/foodborne-germs.html

Chambers KC. Conditioned taste aversions. *World J Otorhinolaryngol Head Neck Surg*. 2018;4(1):92-100. doi: 10.1016/j.wjorl.2018.02.003. PMID: 30035267; PMCID: PMC6051479.

Children's Health. Eight facts about food allergies in children. Children's Health website. Accessed December 16, 2022. https://www.childrens.com/health-wellness/8-facts-about-food-allergies-in-children

Cohut M. How common are food allergies, really? *Medical News Today*. Published January 6, 2019. Accessed December 16, 2022. https://www.medicalnewstoday.com/articles/324094

Collins L, Halmos E. A FODMAP gentle approach. Monash University website.

Published February 24, 2020. Accessed October 12, 2020. https://www.monash-fodmap.com/blog/gentle-fodmap-diet

Cox L, Larenas-Linnemann D, Lockey RF, Passalacqua G. Speaking the same language: The World Allergy Organization subcutaneous immunotherapy systemic reaction grading system. *J Allergy Clin Immunol*. 2010;125(3):569-74, 574.e1-574.e7. doi: 10.1016/j.jaci.2009.10.060. Epub 2010 Feb 7. PMID: 20144472

Cox L, Williams B, Sicherer S, et al. American College of Allergy, Asthma and Immunology Test Task Force; American Academy of Allergy, Asthma and Immunology Specific IgE Test Task Force. Pearls and pitfalls of allergy diagnostic testing: report from the American College of Allergy, Asthma and Immunology/ American Academy of Allergy, Asthma and Immunology Specific IgE Test Task Force. *Ann Allergy Asthma Immunol*. 2008;101(6):580-92. PMID: 19119701.

Crowe SE. Food allergy vs food intolerance in patients with irritable bowel syndrome. *Gastroenterol Hepatol*. 2019;15(1):38-40. PMID: 30899207; PMCID: PMC6423694. https://www.gastroenterologyandhepatology.net/archives/january-2019/food-allergy-vs-food-intolerance-in-patients-with-irritable-bowel-syndrome/)

Drake, L, editor. Hot sauce, wine and tomatoes cause flare-ups, survey finds. Rosacea website. Updated 2005. Accessed December 8, 2021. https://www.rosacea.org/rosacea-review/2005/fall/hot-sauce-wine-and-tomatoes-cause-flare-ups-survey-finds Fall 2005.

Du Toit G, Katz Y, Sasieni P, et al. Early consumption of peanuts in infancy is associated with a low prevalence of peanut allergy. *J Allergy Clin Immunol*. 2008;122(5):984-91. doi: 10.1016/j.jaci.2008.08.039. PMID: 19000582.

Feuille E, Nowak-Węgrzyn A. Food protein-induced enterocolitis syndrome, allergic proctocolitis, and enteropathy. *Curr Allergy Asthma Rep*. 2015;15(8):50. doi: 10.1007/s11882-015-0546-9. PMID: 26174434.

Fonacier L. A practical guide to patch testing. *J Allergy Clin Immunol Pract*. 2015;3(5):669-75. doi: 10.1016/j.jaip.2015.05.001. Epub 2015 Jun 6. PMID: 26054552.

Food Allergy Research & Education. Facts and statistics. Food Allergy Research & Education website. Updated June 4, 2020. Accessed August 25, 2022. https://www.foodallergy.org/resources/facts-and-statistics

Fritzsching B, Contoli M, Porsbjerg C, et al. Freemantle N. Long-term real-world effectiveness of allergy immunotherapy in patients with allergic rhinitis and asthma: results from the REACT study, a retrospective cohort study. *Lancet Reg Health Eur*. 2021;13:100275. doi: 10.1016/j.lanepe.2021.100275. PMID: 34901915; PMCID: PMC8640513.

Fu L, Freedman-Kalchma T, Betchel S, and Sussman G. Diagnosis and treatment of the various types of angioedema. Review of hereditary angioedema. *LymphoSign Journal*. 3(2): 47-53 https://doi.org/10.14785/lymphosign-2016-0001

Gradman J, Halken S. Preventive effect of allergen immunotherapy on asthma and new sensitizations. *J Allergy Clin Immunol Pract*. 2021; 9 (5): 1813-1817. Doi: 10.1016/j.jaip.2021.03.010. Epub 2021 Mar 19. PMID: 33746088.

Gupta RS, Lau CH, Sita EE, et al. Factors associated with reported food allergy tolerance among U.S. children. *Ann Allergy Asthma Immunol*. 2013;111(3):194-198. e4. doi: 10.1016/j.anai.2013.06.026. Epub 2013 Jul 24. PMID: 23987195.

Gupta RS, Warren CM, Smith BM, et al. The public health impact of parent-reported childhood food allergies in the United States. *Pediatrics*. 2018;142(6):e20181235. doi: 10.1542/peds.2018-1235. Epub 2018 Nov 19. Erratum in: Pediatrics. 2019 Mar;143(3): PMID: 30455345; PMCID: PMC6317772.

Gupta RS, Warren CM, Smith BM, et al. Prevalence and severity of food allergies among U.S. adults. *JAMA Netw Open*. 2019;2(1):e185630. doi: 10.1001/jamanetworkopen.2018.5630. PMID: 30646188; PMCID: PMC6324316.

Hayat M, Ali IA, Nusrat S. Emergency department visits and inpatient admissions - trends in IBS over a decade: 439. *Am J Gastroenterol*. 2018;113(S256). DOI:10.14309/00000434-201810001-00439

Hébert JR, Shivappa N, Wirth MD, et al. Perspective: Perspective: The dietary inflammatory index (DII)—lessons learned, improvements made, and future directions. *Adv Nutr*. 2019;10(2):185-195. doi: 10.1093/advances/nmy071. PMID: 30615051; PMCID: PMC6416047.

Hinderliter CF, Goodhart M, Anderson M, Misanin JR. Extended lowered body temperature increases the effective CS-US interval in conditioned taste aversion for adult rats. *Psychol Rep*. 2002;90(3 Pt 1):800-2. doi: 10.2466/pr0.2002.90.3.800. PMID: 12090509.

Horvath K, Perman JA. Autism and gastrointestinal symptoms. *Curr Gastroenterol Rep*. 2002;4(3):251-8. doi: 10.1007/s11894-002-0071-6. PMID: 12010627.

Jensen ET, Martin CF, Kappelman MD, Dellon ES. Prevalence of eosinophilic gastritis, gastroenteritis, and colitis: estimates from a national administrative database. *J Pediatr Gastroenterol Nutr*. 2016;62(1):36-42. doi: 10.1097/MPG.0000000000000865. PMID: 25988554; PMCID: PMC4654708

Kaplan AP, Greaves M. Pathogenesis of chronic urticaria. *Clin Exp Allergy*. 2009;39(6):777-87. doi: 10.1111/j.1365-2222.2009.03256.x. Epub 2009 Apr 22. PMID: 19400905.

Kapur S, Watson W, Carr S. Atopic dermatitis. *Allergy Asthma Clin Immunol*. 201812;14(Suppl 2):52. doi: 10.1186/s13223-018-0281-6. PMID: 30275844; PMCID: PMC6157251.

Kelso JM. Unproven diagnostic tests for adverse reactions to foods. *J Allergy Clin Immunol Pract*. 2018;6(2):362-365. doi: 10.1016/j.jaip.2017.08.021. PMID: 29524991.

Kenawy HI, Boral I, Bevington A. Complement-coagulation cross-talk: a potential mediator of the physiological activation of complement by low pH. *Front*

Immunol. 2015;6:215. doi: 10.3389/fimmu.2015.00215. PMID: 25999953; PMCID: PMC4422095.

Kim H, Fischer D. Anaphylaxis. *Allergy Asthma Clin Immunol*. 2011;7(Suppl 1):S6. doi: 10.1186/1710-1492-7-S1-S6. PMID: 22166113; PMCID: PMC3245439.

Khan SJ, Dharmage SC, Matheson MC, Gurrin LC. Is the atopic march related to confounding by genetics and early-life environment? A systematic review of sibship and twin data. *Allergy*. 2018;73(1):17-28. doi: 10.1111/all.13228. Epub 2017 Jul 12. PMID: 28618023.

Kim BE, Leung DYM. Significance of skin barrier dysfunction in atopic dermatitis. *Allergy Asthma Immunol Res*. 2018;10(3):207-215. doi: 10.4168/aair.2018.10.3.207. PMID: 29676067; PMCID: PMC5911439.

Koch JP, Donaldson RM Jr. A survey of food intolerances in hospitalized patients. *N Engl J Med*. 1964; 24;271:657-60. doi: 10.1056/NEJM196409242711304. PMID: 14170845.

Liu AH, Zeiger RS, Sorkness CS, et al. The Childhood Asthma Control Test: Retrospective determination and clinical validation of a cut point to identify children with very poorly controlled asthma. *J Allergy Clin Immunol 2010;* 126: 267-73.

Liu L. Hereditary angioedema. Kallikrein-bradykinin pathway. October 10, 2019. https://step1.medbullets.com/immunology/105011/hereditary-angioedema

Lyall K, Van de Water J, Ashwood P, Hertz-Picciotto I. Asthma and allergies in children with autism spectrum disorders: results from the CHARGE study. *Autism Res*. 2015;8(5):567-74. doi: 10.1002/aur.1471. Epub 2015 Feb 26. PMID: 25722050; PMCID: PMC6900397.

Maggio E. Polysorbates, biotherapeutics, and anaphylaxis: a review. BioProcess International website. Published September 19, 2017. Accessed December 16, 2022. https://bioprocessintl.com/manufacturing/formulation/polysorbates-biotherapeutics-and-anaphylaxis-a-review/

Maintz L, Novak N. Histamine and histamine intolerance. *Am J Clin Nutr*. 2007;85(5):1185-96. doi: 10.1093/ajcn/85.5.1185. PMID: 17490952. Accessed January 5, 2021

Mali S, Jambure R. Anaphyllaxis management: Current concepts. Anesth Essays Res. 2012;6(2):115-23. https://www.ncbi.nlm.nih.gov/pmc/articles/PMC4173449/ doi: 10.4103/0259-1162.108284. PMID: 25885603; PMCID: PMC4173449.

Massara, EJ, ed. Handbook of human toxicology. 1997. CRC Press. p332.

McGregor MC, Krings JG, Nair P, Castro M. Role of biologics in asthma. *Am J Respir Crit Care Med*. 2019;199(4):433-445. doi: 10.1164/rccm.201810-1944CI. PMID: 30525902; PMCID: PMC6835092. Accessed December 2, 2021.

Medline Plus (National Library of Medicine). Oats. 2021. Updated March 29, 2022. Accessed December 15, 2021. https://medlineplus.gov.

Mennini M, Fiocchi AG, Cafarotti A, et al. Food protein-induced allergic proctocolitis in infants: Literature review and proposal of a management protocol. *World Allergy Organ J*. 2020;13(10):100471. doi: 10.1016/j.waojou.2020.100471. PMID: 33072241; PMCID: PMC7549143

Merle NS, Church SE, Fremeaux-Bacchi V, Roumenina LT. Complement system part I: molecular mechanisms of activation and regulation. *Front Immunol*. 2015;2(6):262. doi: 10.3389/fimmu.2015.00262. PMID: 26082779; PMCID: PMC4451739.

Merle NS, Noe R, Halbwachs-Mecarelli L, Fremeaux-Bacchi V, Roumenina LT. Complement system part II: role in immunity. *Front Immunol*. 2015;6:257:1-26. doi: 10.3389/fimmu.2015.00257. PMID: 26074922; PMCID: PMC4443744.

Molendijk M, Molero P, Ortuño Sánchez-Pedreño F, et al. Diet quality and depression risk: A systematic review and dose-response meta-analysis of prospective studies. *J Affect Disord*. 2018;226:346-354. doi: 10.1016/j.jad.2017.09.022. Epub 2017 Sep 23. PMID: 29031185.

Monsbakken KW, Vandvik PO, Farup PG. Perceived food intolerance in subjects with irritable bowel syndrome--etiology, prevalence and consequences. *Eur J Clin Nutr*. 2006;60(5):667-72. doi: 10.1038/sj.ejcn.1602367. PMID: 16391571.

Moorman JE, Rudd RA, Johnson CA, et al.; Centers for Disease Control and Prevention (CDC). National surveillance for asthma--United States, 1980-2004. *MMWR Surveill Summ*. 2007;56(8):1-54. PMID: 17947969. https://www.cdc.gov/mmwr/preview/mmwrhtml/ss5608a1.htm

Moreau ME, Garbacki N, Molinaro G, Brown NJ, Marceau F, Adam A. The kallikrein-kinin system: current and future pharmacological targets. *J Pharmacol Sci*. 2005;99(1):6-38. doi: 10.1254/jphs.srj05001x. PMID: 16177542.

Morgan Griffin R., Allergy statistics and facts. WebMD website. Updated December 12, 2021. Accessed August 25, 2022. https://www.webmd.com/allergies/allergy-statistics.

Nance CL, Deniskin R, Diaz VC, et al. The role of the microbiome in food allergy: a review. Children (Basel). 2020;7(6):50. doi: 10.3390/children7060050. PMID: 32466620; PMCID: PMC7346163;

National Heart, Lung, and Blood Institute. Asthma management guidelines: focused updates 2021. NHLBI website. Updated February 4, 2021. Accessed December 12, 2021. https://www.nhlbi.nih.gov/health-topics/asthma-management-guidelines-2020-updates

National Heart, Lung, and Blood Institute. National asthma education and prevention program expert panel report 3; guidelines for diagnosis and management of asthma. 2007:1-417. NHLBI website. Updated September, 2012. Accessed December 12, 2021. https://www.nhlbi.nih.gov/health-topics/guidelines-for-diagnosis-management-of-asthma

National Toxicology Program. NTP 12th report on carcinogens. *Rep Carcinog*.

2011;12:iii-499. Accessed December 4-9, 2021. https://monographs.iarc.who. int/ PMID: 21822324.

Nowak-Wegrzyn A, Assa'ad AH, Bahna SL, et al. Adverse reactions to food committee of American Academy of Allergy, Asthma & Immunology. work group report: oral food challenge testing. *J Allergy Clin Immunol*. 2009;123(6 Suppl):S365-83. doi: 10.1016/j.jaci.2009.03.042. PMID: 19500710.

Nowak-Wegrzyn A, Warren CM, Brown-Whitehorn T, et al. Food protein-induced enterocolitis syndrome in the US population-based study. *J Allergy Clin Immunol*. 2019;144(4):1128-1130. doi: 10.1016/j.jaci.2019.06.032. Epub 2019 Jul 6. PMID: 31288044; PMCID: PMC7923683

Nurmagambetov T, Kuwahara R, Garbe P. The economic burden of asthma in the United States, 2008-2013. *Ann Am Thorac Soc*. 2018;15(3):348-356. doi: 10.1513/AnnalsATS.201703-259OC. PMID: 29323930.

Nzeako UC. Diagnosis and management of angioedema with abdominal involvement: a gastroenterology perspective. *World J Gastroenterol*. 2010;16(39):4913-21. doi: 10.3748/wjg.v16.i39.4913. PMID: 20954277; PMCID: PMC2957599.

Orphanet. Search engine for rare disease. Orpha Code-99932 in search term "Heiner's Syndrome" //www.orpha.net/consor/cgi-bin/Disease_Search.php?lng=EN

Pappas A. The relationship of diet and acne: A review. *Dermatoendocrinol*. 2009;1(5):262-7. doi: 10.4161/derm.1.5.10192. PMID: 20808513; PMCID: PMC2836431.

Penagos M, Durham SR. Allergen immunotherapy for long-term tolerance and prevention. *J Allergy Clin Immunol*. 2022;149(3):802-811. doi: 10.1016/j.jaci.2022.01.007. Epub 2022 Jan 24. PMID: 35085663.

Picco MF. Celiac disease diet: how do I get enough grains? Mayo Clinic website. N.D. Accessed December 15, 2021.

Pimentel M, Lembo A. Microbiome and its role in irritable bowel syndrome. *Dig Dis Sci*. 2020;65(3):829-839. doi: 10.1007/s10620-020-06109-5. PMID: 32026278. ;

Pinczower GD, Bertalli NA, Bussmann N, et al. The effect of provision of an adrenaline autoinjector on quality of life in children with food allergy. *J Allergy Clin Immunol*. 2013131(1):238-40.e1. doi: 10.1016/j.jaci.2012.09.038. Epub 2012 Nov 27. PMID: 23199601.

Radke TJ, Brown LG, Faw B, et al. Restaurant food allergy practices - six selected sites, United States, 2014. *MMWR Morb Mortal Wkly Rep*. 2017;66(15):404-407. doi: 10.15585/mmwr.mm6615a2. PMID: 28426639; PMCID: PMC5687189.

Raiten DJ. Nutrition and pharmacology: general principles and implications for HIV. *Am J Clin Nutr*. 2011;94(6):1697S-1702S. doi: 10.3945/ajcn.111.019109. Epub 2011 Nov 16. PMID: 22089445; PMCID: PMC3225603.

Rasmussen ER, Mey K, Bygum A. Angiotensin-converting enzyme inhibitor-induced angioedema--a dangerous new epidemic. *Acta Derm Venereol*. 2014;94(3):260-4. doi: 10.2340/00015555-1760. PMID: 24285044.

Reddel HK, Bacharier LB, Bateman ED, et al. Global initiative for asthma strategy 2021: executive summary and rationale for key changes. *Eur Respir J*. 2021;59(1):2102730. doi: 10.1183/13993003.02730-2021. PMID: 34667060; PMCID: PMC8719459.

Rubio-Tapia A, Hill ID, Kelly CP, et al. American College of Gastroenterology. ACG clinical guidelines: diagnosis and management of celiac disease. *Am J Gastroenterol*. 2013;108(5):656-76; quiz 677. doi: 10.1038/ajg.2013.79. Epub 2013 Apr 23. PMID: 23609613; PMCID: PMC3706994.

Ryder E. Pollen-food allergy syndrome. Dermnetnz website. Published January, 2018. Updated May 2021. Accessed November 5, 2022. https://dermnetnz.org/topics/pollen-food-allergy-syndrome

Salazar A, Velázquez-Soto H, Ayala-Balboa J, Jiménez-Martínez MC. Allergen-based diagnostic: novel and old methodologies with new approaches. In: Athari SS, ed. *Allergen*. InTech; 2017. Books. https://www.intechopen.com/chapters/55713; 2017, October 4th; doi: 10.5772/intechopen.69276; accessed 12/07/2021.

Sampson HA, Aceves S, Bock SA, et al. Food allergy: a practice parameter update-2014. *J Allergy Clin Immunol*. 2014;134(5):1016-25.e43. doi: 10.1016/j.jaci.2014.05.013. Epub 2014 Aug 28. PMID: 25174862.

Schatz M, Sorkness CA, Li JT, et al.. Asthma control test: reliability, validity, and responsiveness in patients not previously followed by asthma specialists. *J Allergy Clin Immunol*. 2006;117(3):549-56. doi: 10.1016/j.jaci.2006.01.011. PMID: 16522452.

Sethi TJ, Lessof MH, Kemeny DM, et al. How reliable are commercial allergy tests? *Lancet*. 1987;1(8524):92-4. doi: 10.1016/s0140-6736(87)91922-2. PMID: 2879187.

Shivappa N, Steck SE, Hurley TG, Hussey JR, Hébert JR. Designing and developing a literature-derived, population-based dietary inflammatory index. *Public Health Nutr*. 2014;17(8):1689-96. doi: 10.1017/S1368980013002115. Epub 2013 Aug 14. PMID: 23941862; PMCID: PMC3925198.

Sicherer SH, Sampson HA. Food allergy. *J Allergy Clin Immunol*. 2010;125(2 Suppl 2):S116-25. doi: 10.1016/j.jaci.2009.08.028. Epub 2009 Dec 29. PMID: 20042231.

Smith M. Another person's poison. *Lancet*. 2014;384(9959):2019-20. doi: 10.1016/s0140-6736(14)62327-8. PMID: 25489647.

Staller K, Olén O, Söderling J, et al. Mortality risk in irritable bowel syndrome: results from a nationwide prospective cohort study. *Am J Gastroenterol*. 2020;115(5):746-755. doi: 10.14309/ajg.0000000000000573. PMID: 32108661; PMCID: PMC7196022.

Steck SE, Shivappa N, Tabung FK, et al. The dietary inflammatory index: a new tool for assessing diet quality based on inflammatory potential. *The Digest*. 2014;49(1-9). https://www.researchgate.net/publication/264554956_The_Dietary_

Inflammatory_Index_A_New_Tool_for_Assessing_Diet_Quality_Based_on_Inflammatory_Potential/citation/download

Sunkara T, Rawla P, Yarlagadda KS, Gaduputi V. Eosinophilic gastroenteritis: diagnosis and clinical perspectives. *Clin Exp Gastroenterol*. 2019;12:239-253. doi: 10.2147/CEG.S173130. PMID: 31239747; PMCID: PMC6556468.

Tuano KS, Orange JS, Sullivan K, et al. Food allergy in patients with primary immunodeficiency diseases: prevalence within the US Immunodeficiency Network (USIDNET). *J Allergy Clin Immunol*. 2015;135(1):273-5. doi: 10.1016/j.jaci.2014.09.024. Epub 2014 Nov 25. Erratum in: *J Allergy Clin Immunol*. 2015;135(4):1092. Erratum in: *J Allergy Clin Immunol*. 2015;135(4):1092. PMID: 25441296; PMCID: PMC4324505.

U. S. Department of Health and Human Services. National Institute of Diabetes and Digestive Diseases and Kidney Diseases (NIDDK). Celiac disease testing. NIDDK website. Updated February, 2021. Accessed December 15, 2021. https://www.niddk.nih.gov/health-information/professionals/clinical-tools-patient-management/digestive-diseases/celiac-disease-health-care-professionals

Unsworth DJ, Lock RJ. Food allergy testing. *Adv Clin Chem*. 2014;65:173-98. doi: 10.1016/b978-0-12-800141-7.00006-1. PMID: 25233614.

van Sadelhoff JHJ, Perez Pardo P, Wu J, et al. The gut-immune-brain axis in autism spectrum disorders; a focus on amino acids. *Front Endocrinol* (Lausanne). 2019;10:247. doi: 10.3389/fendo.2019.00247. PMID: 31057483; PMCID: PMC6477881.

Wang, J, Jones, SM, Pongracic, JA, et al. The effect of provision of an adrenaline autoinjector on quality of life in children with food allergy. *J Allergy Clin Immunol*. 2013;131(1):238-241.e1.

Warren CM, Chadha AS, Sicherer SH, et al. Prevalence and severity of sesame allergy in the United States. *JAMA Netw Open*. 2019;2(8):e199144. doi: 10.1001/jamanetworkopen.2019.9144. PMID: 31373655; PMCID: PMC6681546.

Weiss E, Katta R. Diet and rosacea: the role of dietary change in the management of rosacea. *Dermatol Pract Concept*. 2017;7(4):31-37. doi: 10.5826/dpc.0704a08. PMID: 29214107; PMCID: PMC5718124.

World Health Organization. Healthy diet. World Health Organization website. Updated April 29, 2020. Accessed December 8, 2021. https://www.who.int/news-room/fact-sheets/detail/healthy-diet.

Xu G, Snetselaar LG, Jing J, Liu B, Strathearn L, Bao W. Association of food allergy, other allergies with autism spectrum disorder in children. *JAMA Netw Open*. 2018;1(2):e180279. doi: 10.1001/jamanetworkopen.2018.0279. PMID: 30646068; PMCID: PMC6324407.

Yaghoubi M, Adibi A, Safari A, FitzGerald JM, Sadatsafavi M. The projected economic and health burden of uncontrolled asthma in the United States. *Am J Respir Crit*

Care Med. 2019;200(9):1102-1112. doi: 10.1164/rccm.201901-0016OC. PMID: 31166782; PMCID: PMC6888652.

Yu, C, Tang, H, Guo, Y, et al. Hot tea consumption and its interactions with alcohol and tobacco use on the risk for esophageal cancer. *Ann Intern Med.* 2018;168(7):489-497. doi: 10.7326/M17-2000. Epub 2018 Feb 6. Erratum in: *Ann Intern Med.* 2018 May 1;168(9):684. PMID: 29404576; PMCID: PMC6675598.

Zhang, L., Zeng, X., Guo, D. *et al.* Early use of probiotics might prevent antibiotic-associated diarrhea in elderly (>65 years): a systematic review and meta-analysis. *BMC Geriatr.* 2022;22(1):562. doi: 10.1186/s12877-022-03257-3. PMID: 35794520; PMCID: PMC9260993

Reference List for Figures

Figure 1. BioProcess International website. Published September 19, 2017. Accessed December 16, 2022. https://bioprocessintl.com/manufacturing/formulation/polysorbates-biotherapeutics-and-anaphylaxis-a-review/

Figure 2. Adapted from stock image 1057942834. ©iStock.com/Good_Stock. Published October 23, 2018. Purchased October 18, 2022.

Figure 3. Adapted from stock image 111396095. ©iStock.com/Good_Stock. Published October 23, 2018. Purchased October 18, 2022.

Figure 4. Adapted from Cox L, Larenas-Linnemann D, Lockey RF, Passalacqua G. Speaking the same language: The World Allergy Organization Subcutaneous Immunotherapy Systemic Reaction Grading System. *J Allergy Clin Immunol*. 2010;125:569-74, 74 e1-74 e7

Figure 6. Steps of Anaphylaxis. Adapted from Maggio E. Polysorbates, biotherapeutics, and anaphylaxis: a review.

Figure 8. Adapted from image https://www.benaroyaresearch.org/sites/default/files/bio-8-top-allergies-550w.jpg

Figure 12. Adapted from Salazar, A, Velázquez-Soto, H, and Jiménez-Martínez, JA. Allergen-based diagnostic: novel and old methodologies with new approaches. In (Ed.), *Allergen*. IntechOpen. Published October 4, 2017. Accessed December 7, 2021. https://doi.org/10.5772/intechopen.69276

Figure 23. Adapted from What is celiac disease? Figure 1. https://www.beyondceliac.org/celiac-disease

Figure 27. Adapted from Fu LW, Freedman-Kalchman T, Betchel S, Sussman G. Review of hereditary angioedema. *LymphoSign Journal*. Published May 10, 2016;3:47-53. https://lymphosign.com/doi/10.14785/lymphosign-2016-0001

Figure 29. Adapted from Illustration Pathology of Asthma Editable Word Template #03975. https://www.editabletemplates.com/download-microsoft-word-templates/illustration-pathology-of-asthma-editable-word-template-3975.html

Figures 30 and 31. Childrens' Asthma Control Test (C-ACT) permission to use granted by: Mapi Research Trust, Lyon, France, https://eprovide.mapi-trust.org. 2002 QualityMetric, Inc. Asthma Control Test is a trademark of QualityMetric Incorporated.

Figures 30 and 31. Liu AH, Zeiger RS, Sorkness CS, et al. The Childhood Asthma Control Test: Retrospective determination and clinical validation of a cut point to identify children with very poorly controlled asthma. J Allergy Clin Immunol 2010; 12 6: 267-73.

Figure 32. Adapted from stock image 1057941320. ©iStock.com/Good_Stock. Published October 23, 2018. Purchased October 18, 2022.

Figure 33. Adapted from Ryder E. Pollen-food allergy syndrome. Dermnetnz website. Published January, 2018. Updated May 2021. Accessed November 5, 2022. https://dermnetnz.org/topics/pollen-food-allergy-syndrome

Figure 41. Contact dermatitis of the palms. Adapted from Oakley, A. What Does Contact Dermatitis Look Like? 2012. Accessed November 1, 2022. https://dermnetnz.org/topics/contact-dermatitis

Figure 52. Adapted from stock image 253085703 ©Yomogi1/Dreamstime.com. Purchased January 10, 2023.

Figure 56. Images reproduced with permission from Monash University (monashfodmap.com) Department of Gastroenterology, Monash University. Images reproduced with permission from Monash University (monashfodmap.com). Download the Monash University FODMAP Diet App for a comprehensive food guide containing the FODMAP ratings and serving sizes for hundreds of different foods and beverages. Available on iOS and Android.

Figure 57. Illustration of Bristol Stool Scale. Adapted from Rome IV Criteria. Appendix A: Rome IV Diagnostic Criteria for FGIDs. Diagnostic criteria for IBS subtypes. January 16, 2016. Accessed October 1, 2022. https://theromefoundation.org/rome-iv/rome-iv-criteria/

Figure 60. Adapted from Steck, SE, Shivappa, N, Tabung, F, et al. The dietary inflammatory index: a new tool for assessing diet quality based on inflammatory potential. *The Digest*. July, 2014;49(1-9).

Review Inquiry

Hey, it's Julie here.

I hope you've enjoyed the book, finding it both useful and fun. I have a favor to ask you.

Would you consider giving it a rating wherever you bought the book? Online book stores are more likely to promote a book when they feel good about its content, and reader reviews are a great barometer for a book's quality.

So please go to the website of wherever you bought the book, search for my name and the book title, and leave a review. If able, perhaps consider adding a picture of you holding the book. That increases the likelihood your review will be accepted!

Many thanks in advance,
Julie Wendt

Will You Share the Love?

Get this book for a friend, associate, or family member!

If you have found this book valuable and know others who would find it useful, consider buying them a copy as a gift. Special bulk discounts for 25+ copies are available if you would like your whole team or organization to benefit from reading *What's Eating Our Kids? A Parent's Guide to Food Allergy, Intolerance, and Toxicity*.

Learn more at: www.relieveallergyaz.com/book

Would You Like Dr. Julie Wendt to Speak to Your Organization?

Book Julie Now!

Dr. Julie Wendt accepts a limited number of speaking and training engagements each year. To learn how you can bring her message to your organization, email her at: bookjulie@relieveaz.com.

About the Author

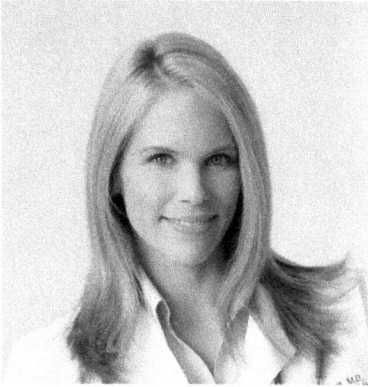

Julie Wendt, MD, FACAAI, FAAAAI, FACP, DABOM

Dr. Wendt earned Bachelor of Science degrees with honors in biochemistry and biology from the University of Illinois, a degree in microbiology and immunology from Vanderbilt University and a Doctor of Medicine degree from the University of Tennessee College of Medicine. She completed a residency in Internal Medicine and an Allergy and Immunology fellowship at Rush University Medical Center in Chicago.

In private practice since 2005, Dr. Wendt has published a great deal of research. She has received the American Medical Association Physician's Recognition Award, a Patient's Choice Award, and is noted as one of America's Top Physicians. Dr. Wendt is former President of the Arizona Allergy and Asthma Society.

A native of Chicago, Dr. Wendt is married to Philip Bach, a Nebraskan. They have seven children, ages 12 to 29. She enjoys fencing, boating, water skiing, scuba diving, and traveling. In her free time, Dr. Wendt enjoys serving with multiple charitable organizations including Global Orphan Project and Family Promise.

FACAAI – Fellow of the American College of Allergy, Asthma & Immunology
FAAAAI – Fellow of the American Academy of Allergy, Asthma & Immunology
FACP – Fellow of the American College of Physicians
DABOM – Diplomat of the American Board of Obesity Medicine

Dr. Wendt can be reached at: bookjulie@relieveaz.com